The Essential Keto Vegan Cookbook And Lifestyle For Beginners

The Complete Low Carb, Plant Based Recipe Diet Guide For Weight Loss, Reverse Disease And Boost Brain Health

Kylie Benson

Table Of Contents

Day Two, Breakfast

    Avocado Toast- Bread Recipe 1

Day Two, Lunch

    Turmeric & Cauliflower Soup

Day Two, Dinner

    Veggie Pizza

Day Two, Snack

    Cinnamon Trail Mix

Day Three, Breakfast

    Protein Smoothie- Vanilla Almond

Day Three, Lunch

    Tortilla Recipe- Fajitas

Day Three, Dinner

Creamy Vegetable Stir Fry

Day Three, Snack

    Fat Bomb- Pecan Dream

Day Four, Breakfast

    Cinnamon Roll Pancakes

Day Four, Lunch

    Greek Salad- Vegan Cheese Recipe

Day Four, Dinner

    Spaghetti with Homemade Sauce

Day Four, Snack

    Chocolate Ice Cream

Day Five, Breakfast

    English Muffin and Eggs

Day Five, Lunch

    Chili

Day Five, Dinner

    Portobello Burgers

Day Five, Snack

Day Nine, Snack

    Carrot Cake Bites

Day Ten, Breakfast

    Overnight Oats

Day Ten, Lunch

    Egg Salad

Day Ten, Dinner

    Falafel

Day Ten, Snack

    Candied Nuts

Day Eleven, Breakfast

    Breakfast Smoothie- Strawberry

Day Eleven, Lunch

    Tomato Soup

Day Eleven, Dinner

    Grilled Portobello with Spinach

Day Eleven, Snack

    Zucchini Chips- Taco Seasoning Recipe

Day Twelve, Breakfast

    Bagel

Day Twelve, Lunch

    Fajita Salad- Sour Cream Recipe

Day Twelve, Dinner

    Buffalo Bites

Day Twelve, Snack

    Coconut Clusters

Day Thirteen, Breakfast

    Chocolate Pudding

Day Thirteen, Lunch

    Pasta Salad

Day Thirteen, Dinner

Introduction

With so many options and diets being advertised, knowing the right way to stay healthy has become confusing. Researching which diet is best, or which exercise program will shed the most pounds, has become tiresome. With endless food options, and restaurant chains on every corner, staying fit and healthy has become more challenging than ever. As technology advances, so does the research on different foods and lifestyles.

With the world population ever growing, new challenges also arise to feed everyone sustainably. The health of our bodies, the environment, and the treatment of animals are on the decline. Unlike before, foods and animals are being injected with chemicals, unhealthy fats, and tons of sugar to preserve food longer and satisfy the high demands of the consumer. Hidden dangers hide in foods once considered healthy.

In the past, refined carbs and extra sugars didn't exist. As manufacturers and giant companies grow, food production changes. This relatively new increase in sugar and refined carbohydrates brings a whole slew of new problems. Obesity, heart disease, diabetes, cancers, physiological diseases, and aging have all exponentially increased over the last decade. So what can be done?

The Ketogenic-Vegan diet is the simple solution. Ketogenic or Keto for short refers to a low carbohydrate and sugar lifestyle. What many don't know is that the human body doesn't need large amounts of carbs to survive. Our bodies are sustainable on their own with the exception of a few vitamins. The human body produces a special type of energy that can only be tapped into with the absence of carbs. This energy is preferred by the body and brain and serves as a more efficient fuel source. When carbs are severely restricted, a compound called ketone bodies are released into the system.

Ketone bodies replace glucose, the energy source produced when carbs are consumed. It's thought that in ancestral times, ketone bodies were used over glucose by the human body. Glucose as a source of energy can be compared to coal or diesel. When put into an automobile both substances are messy, dirty, and leave behind residue. However, ketone bodies can be compared to solar power or electric cars. Both of which run quietly, cleanly, and leave little to no waste. Replacing carbs with fats will lead to the body producing and using the better fuel source with ketone bodies.

The Keto diet requires consuming high amounts of fats that most people aren't used to consuming. A common misconception about consuming high amounts of fat is that fat consumption leads to weight gain. However, many studies have proven this wrong. The keto diet has gained an immense amount of popularity from the general public because of its success with weight loss. There is simple science that can explain why carbs and sugars are the true culprit in weight gain. This guide will discuss those reasons but in summary, carbs trigger a response in insulin and blood sugars within the body.

This spike leads does lead to quick, but unsustained, energy. This triggers an inflammatory response in the body, and food is inevitably stored as body fat. Fats are digested completely differently than carbs. Fat releases slow and sustained energy throughout digestion as it takes longer to break down. Fats do not create an inflammatory effect like carbs and are able to be digested completely.

Following the Keto diet with vegan food will not only aid in weight loss, but will provide numerous health benefits and environmental benefits. Veganism has become popular over the years as more information comes forth on the meat and dairy industry. The industry has grown so large that producing mass amounts of food ethically has become impossible. Quantity over quality is the new method and low quality products are taking a toll on human health, animal rights, and the environment.

Small and local farmers have a hard time competing with large production giants. To keep mass amounts of animal products safe for consumption, chemicals, medicines, and unnatural substances are being injected into animals to help them grow larger, faster. Animals are suffering due to the high demand from a growing population. In addition, more and more land and animals are needed every year to compensate for the shorter life span these stressed, animals endure. In addition, the amount of land needed to produce high quantities of animal products is taking away from other industries and in turn polluting the environment. The meat and dairy industry accounts for an extremely high amount of carbon emissions, which leads to even more problems for the environment. This guide will address many of those problems.

Participating in a vegan diet will protect innocent animals, the environment and your body from disease and cancer. More and more studies have been published regarding the effect animal products have on the human body. Scientific studies can now link meat and dairy to certain cancers and diseases. Specific examples and studies on how animal products affect overall human health will be discussed.

Combining a Keto-Vegan diet will lead to physical and internal changes. Physically, the Keto-Vegan diet will produce a healthy, lean, and toned physique. Better hair, skin, nails and anti-aging effects are all proven benefits of is diet. Not only does the "diet improve physical appearance but internally almost every organ will become healthier. Brain and heart health are significantly impacted by a Keto-Vegan diet. Not only does the diet give protection from certain diseases and cancers, but the Keto-Vegan diet has the ability to change the cellular DNA that determines an individual's lifespan as discussed later in this guide. Mental acuity and higher energy levels are all associated with a Keto-Vegan diet. Studies have shown that overall health increases in almost every aspect, while on a Keto-Vegan diet.

Starting a Keto-Vegan diet is much different than other diets and is simple with this guide. The Keto diet is fat focused and fortunately does not restrict you from eating or feeling starved. Instead of feeling hungry, tired, and unsatisfied like other diets, the body will be full of energy and have a feeling of fullness. Although carbs and sugar are not allowed on a Keto diet, they won't be missed.

One of the best things about this diet is that almost any food can be enjoyed with a few moderations. This guide will give numerous recipes and Keto-Vegan moderations that all mimic a standard, everyday diet. Typical dishes, whether starting this diet as a vegan or not, will give alternatives to animal products like meat and cheese.

Although some may want to cut calories in the beginning to speed up weight loss, a calorie deficit is not needed to be successful on this diet. Reaching macro counts is more important for success. This guide will give you the breakdown of what you should be eating day to day in regards to fats, proteins, and carbs.

Along with starting a Keto-Diet, this guide will explain intermittent fasting and its benefits. Intermittent fasting is a helpful tool that can be implemented into the Keto-Vegan diet. Intermittent fasting allows cells to rejuvenate and be strong while aiding in weight loss. Intermittent fasting is beneficial for just about everyone and this guide will give you all the information you need to get started.

If you're ready to learn the success of the Keto diet and discover the vegan lifestyle, look no further than this guide. This guide gives everything worth knowing about both diets and will help you transition into the combined diet seamlessly. Not only will this guide give proven scientific research surrounding both diets, but we will break the studies down into easy to understand, useful information.

Tips and tricks are included to ensure a smooth transition in the beginning and throughout the lifestyle change. In addition, tons of recipes with your favorite foods are given. You'll learn how to transform your favorite food into a nutritious, healthy, and low carbohydrate meal that will give power and energy to your body. These recipes are all ketogenic and 100% vegan. Each recipe will leave your body feeling satisfied and energized, all while supporting weight loss. If you're ready to dive into this important information, keep reading! Please leave a review if you enjoy the information and recipes in this guide!

Chapter 1: Why the Vegan Lifestyle?

With so much misinformation surrounding the vegan lifestyle, this chapter will tell you everything you need to know, in an unbiased way that's backed by scientific research. Whatever reason led you to embark on the vegan diet, know that your body, animals, and the environment will benefit from your decision.

Veganism 101

Although the term vegan was coined in the 1940's, veganism concepts have been around for over 2000 years. Practices of veganism can be traced back to 500 BCE with the accomplished Greek mathematician and philosopher, Pythagorus. In the same time period Siddhārtha Gautama, also known as Buddha, promoted a vegetarian lifestyle. Later in 1806 CE, eggs and dairy were thought to be unethical as well, regarding the treatment of animals. Fast-forward to 1944, Donald Watson called a meeting with five other non-dairy vegetarians and thus started a new movement. The word vegan was formed and is derived from the first three letters and last two letters of the word vegetarian. The group created a "society" whose main efforts sought to end animal cruelty and exploitation.

In today's world, veganism and vegetarian lifestyles are ever growing. According to the Guardian (2018), one in eight Britons are now vegetarian or vegan. It's estimated that 21% claim to be flexitarian, meaning their consumption of animal products has drastically lessened and these individuals primarily follow a plant based diet (Smithers, 2018). It's estimated that even more people have changed and lessened their consumption of animal products, loosely following a plant based diet.

Supermarket giant Sainsbury recently released a study about the future of food. The report predicts trends in food over the next 150 years. Algae milk lattes and cellular based meat were predicted to be high competitors to animal based products. The report mentions the high increase in recent demand for plant based and vegan products and the report predicts that one in four people with be vegan by 2025 (A Quarter of Brits Will be Vegan by 2025 and Half will be Flexitarian, 2019).

More and more people are becoming aware of how animals are being treated, the positive effects of veganism have on the human body, and how the animal industry is affecting the environment. Although there are numerous reasons to go vegan and eat a plant-based diet, most reasons fall under two categories: health and ethical.

Veganism for Health Purposes

Many chose the vegan lifestyle for health reasons. Whether fighting a disease or already in good health, there are numerous reasons to eliminate animal products from our daily lives. What many don't know is that studies have shown that meat and animal products have a direct effect on body composition, heart disease, cancers, and other illnesses. Choosing the vegan lifestyle not only eliminates many health risks, but fills the body with highly nutritious foods that work with the body to develop perfect health. Below are the main health reasons to choose a vegan diet.

Body Composition and Fitness

Many chose a Keto-Vegan lifestyle to lose weight and maintain a slender physique. Luckily, not only will the Keto-Vegan lifestyle shed weight quicker than any other diet, but it can also transform into a sustainable lifestyle that will keep an individual at a healthy weight. A study by the Journal of the Academy of Nutrition and Dietetics (2013) compared individuals on a meat diet to individuals that were vegan or vegetarian. The study found that the participants on a meat diet consumed far less fiber, plant proteins, and vital nutrients compared to vegans. The study also found that even though the calories between the groups were the same, those consuming a non-vegan diet had the highest body mass index. The subjects in the vegan group averaged a healthy body mass of 24 while those in a non-vegan diet averaged 28.7. This is alarming considering both groups consumed the same amount of calories.

Meat vs. Cancer

Although there are other factors like genetics, exercise, and smoking, that increase the risk for cancer, unhealthy diets also play a prominent role. A healthy, active lifestyle is up to you, and you should start with consuming the right foods. For starters, the vegan diet is filled with healthy vegetables, fruits, nuts, and seeds. All of which contain vital and nutritious properties. Consuming healthy foods will obviously reduce the risk of disease and aid in a healthier lifestyle, but there's a bit more to it.

A study done by Oxford University compared about 60,000 British men and women over a 15-year period. Some of the participants had a meat eating diet while others only consumed vegetarian or vegan foods. When the study concluded, they found that the overall cancer incidence was 11% lower in vegetarians and 19% lower in vegans compared to participants eating a meat filled diet (Key, et al., 2014). The study showed staggering results, especially in regards to vegan diets.

Meat contains many substances that are toxic to the body. Although animals and humans are considered mammals, they're not the same. The metabolic processes and brain function capabilities are completely different. One of the best examples of this statement is the fact that cows have four stomachs. The five most toxic, cancer-causing substances from animals are estrogen, insulin-like growth factor, hydrogen sulfide, heterocyclic amines, and cholesterol. Keep in mind that there is other reasons meat is harmful to health.

One of the most common cancers for women is breast cancer. There are many factors that decide the probability of developing breast cancer. What scientists know is that 80% of all breast cancers grow according to estrogen supply (Brechon, 2013). In fact, estrogen production must be controlled and lowered in order to treat breast cancer. Although scientists aren't sure of the exact mechanisms of how estrogen effects breast cancer, it's agreed upon that Estrogen plays a heavy role. Estrogen is a natural hormone produced in the body, but the problem lies when unnatural forms are consumed from chemicals found in foods. Estrogen from mammals is 10,000 more potent in the human body than all other forms of chemically produced, unnatural estrogen (Aksglaede, et al, 2006).

Insulin-like growth factor or IGF-1 is also found in meats and directly linked to breast cancer, ovarian, prostate, and colorectal cancers (Weroha & Haluska, 2012). Because IGF-1 is essentially found in meat proteins, this is another cancer-causing ingredient found in meat. This compound in high amounts is a problem to the human body because IGF-1 triggers cancer growth to begin with and further feeds cancer cells (Chi, et al, 2000). A study showered that when cancer patients were placed on a vegan diet, their conditions and IGF-1 significantly decreased (Soliman, et al, 2011).

Protein fermentation and hydrogen sulfide production is the third reason why meat is linked to cancer. When protein is consumed from plants, the digestive system is able to fully digest it, without creating any harmful byproducts within the body. Plant proteins are usually broken down by the time they reach the large intestine. When meat is consumed, complete digestion does not occur and proteins then enter the large intestine where fermentation occurs. Fermentation within the human body is not a natural occurrence. Animal proteins contain sulfur and ultimately ferments into hydrogen sulfide in the large intestine. Hydrogen sulfide lets off a rotten-egg like odor and is also known as a genotoxin. A genotoxin can destroy and damage deoxyribonucleic acid or DNA according to a study (Attene-Ramos, et al., 2007). The study showed that as sulfide levels increased, DNA damage increased as a result. Hydrogen sulfide molecules are able to travel throughout the blood, thus making them dangerous to cells in every organ of the body.

When consuming meat products, cooking is usually required. Raw meat is only consumed in rare cases. The fourth reason why meat is linked to cancer is due to the properties formed once exposed to heat. When cooking meat, especially at a high temperature, substances like heterocyclic amines are formed. Heterocyclic amines are known to be carcinogenic and cancer causing (National Research Council (US) Committee on Diet, Nutrition, & Cancer, 1982).

Lastly, red and white meat directly affects levels of cholesterol within the body. The body is fully capable with making healthy levels of cholesterol on its own. The problem lies when unnatural, altered cholesterol enters the body from an animal source. Cholesterol is only found in animal products and is not found in plant products, ever. The effect of cholesterol on cancer has been studied for years. Although most agree that there is a link, the causation cholesterol has on cancer is not yet known. However, the link is still being investigated. A study on mice, for example, showed that scientists could control cancer cells in mice by manipulating the amount of cholesterol within the mouse. The higher the level, the faster and more aggressive the cancer spread (Wang, et al., 2018). Although this study was only done in mice, it is another reason to think consider cutting out animal based products and meat.

Heart Disease

Heart disease is the broader term for many heart related problems. These problems include coronary heart disease, arrhythmia, myocardial infarction, dilated cardiomyopathy and heart failure to name a few. According to the British Heart Foundation or BHF (2019), nearly seven and a half million people are living with heart or circulatory disease in the United Kingdom. This equates to 28% of the current population. Furthermore, heart disease takes 170,000 deaths lives yearly, 45,000 of which are marked as premature (Facts and Figures, 2019). The BHF (2019) states that every five minutes, an individual is admitted to a UK hospital for a heart attack and nine billion Euros are spent on Heart and Circulatory diseases yearly. These numbers are alarming and sadly are growing each year.

One study found a strong correlation between processed meats and certain diseases. The study performed by Harvard School of Public Health explains that eating one hot dog or a few slices of salami daily, increases the risk for heart disease by 42% (Boyles, 2010). Processed meats include bacon, frankfurters, some deli meat, hot dogs, salami, and ham to name a few popular items. In addition, these processed meats are also marked as a Type I carcinogen, known to cause cancer, according to the World Health Organization (2015). In addition, the WHO (2015) also classified other red meat like beef, lamb, and pork as Group 2A carcinogens, which are also linked to cancers. Avoiding meat altogether will not hurt the body and will likely aid in the prevention of heart disease and other cancers.

In addition to protecting the heart, veganism can actually reverse heart disease. One study looked at almost 200 patients who started to consume a plant based diet. The majority of participants were able to report a reduction in symptoms and 22%

experienced disease reversal, confirmed by tests (Can a plant-based diet 'reverse' heart disease, 2018).

Diabetes

Diabetes is a disease where the body's ability to produce or respond to the hormone insulin is impaired. This results in the improper metabolization of carbohydrates and elevated glucose levels in the blood. It's estimated that almost four million people have diabetes in the United Kingdom and that a diabetes diagnosis takes places every two minutes (Facts & Figures, 2019). In the United States over 29 million are suffering from diabetes and research suggests that one out of three adults has prediabetes (Santos-Longhurst, 2019).

Cases of undiagnosed diabetes cost the United States an estimated $245 billion and this number is expected to grow (National Diabetes Statistics Report, 2018). Diabetes triggers feelings of hunger, thirst, blurry vision, fatigue, and numbness along with other health complications. Type two diabetes can cause life-threatening complications like heart disease, stroke, nerve damage, neuropathy, kidney disease, and vision problems. Diabetes can be brought on by a sedentary lifestyle, unhealthy diet, family history, and aging within the body.

A Keto-Vegan diet works to maintain healthy blood sugar levels by eliminating unhealthy carbs, refined sugars, and animal products. According to a study, a higher intake of red meat and poultry significantly increased the risk of developing diabetes due to the higher content of heme iron found in meats (Eating Meat Linked to Higher Risk of Disease, 2017). In addition, studies have found that plant based diets are highly effective in the reversal of diabetes, and many are able to discontinue medications (Coote & Sadeghi MD, 2017). Eating a plant-based, vegan diet also allows more vitamins, minerals, and fiber to be present in the body. Fiber is an important component to blood sugar levels and is often deficient in meat heavy diets. Obtaining the right nutrients and cutting out animal products will keep or transform the body to it's healthiest state.

Nutritional Foods

When consuming a vegan diet, almost every single food holds high nutritional value. A plant-based diet is wholesome, earth grown food that contains essential vitamins and minerals. The healthiest, super foods of the world all fall into the vegan category. The term "super food" has been coined over the years and categorizes foods that hold the highest level of nutrition per calorie. Although the order of this list is subjective due to different nutrients in each food, generally super food lists agree with one another.

The top accepted super foods are dark leafy greens, berries, green tea, legumes, nuts, seeds, garlic, olive oil, ginger, turmeric, avocado, sweet potatoes, mushrooms, and seaweed. Notice that each food is produced by nature. When consuming a vegan diet, each meal is filled with foods holding high nutrition and contains essential antioxidants, vitamins, and minerals that can't be found elsewhere.

Antioxidants play a key role in cellular health. Antioxidants protect cells from damage that comes from free radicals. Free radicals naturally form in the body after being exposed to cigarettes, air pollutants, or toxic chemicals. Free radicals have the ability to harm DNA and the structures within cells. Free radicals enhance the aging process within the body by causing oxidative stress. In addition, accumulated oxidative stress is linked to other health problems and certain cancers. According to Healthline author Ryan Raman who holds a Master's in Nutrition & Dietetics and is a registered dietician, the foods containing the highest amount of antioxidants include cocoa, pecans, blueberries, strawberries, artichokes, goji berries, raspberries, kale, red cabbage, beans, beets, and spinach (Raman, 2018). Interestingly, notice the top twelve foods mentioned are all considered vegan. Consuming foods with antioxidants will reduce the risk of disease and keep the body healthy.

Live a Longer, Happier Life
One of the keys to a healthy, long life lies in DNA. DNA is packaged into thin, thread-like structures and live within the nucleus of a cell. Specifically, these threads of DNA are called chromosomes. At the end of each chromosome lie telomeres. Telomeres can be compared to the plastic on the end of a shoe lake. The plastic prevents the ends of the shoelace from fraying. Telomeres are similar and protect chromosomes and DNA from fraying or sticking to each other. Studies have shown that telomeres and their length correlate with an individual's lifespan.
Over time, DNA divides and separates into new chromosomes, which in turn lead to the shortening of telomeres. This is because when new chromosomes are formed, telomeres go with it. When telomeres shorten, less gene expression occurs. This is the process of aging where genes become harder to utilize and harder to repair. When a healthy baby is born, telomeres are at their best and can divide and repair with strength. As this process occurs over time, telomeres get shorter and shorter and have a hard time protecting the DNA wrapped around each chromosome. When this occurs, cells become weaker and unable to function like they once had.

Scientists have been studying telomeres for years to figure out how to preserve them and reverse aging outwardly and within the body. There are known factors that shortened telomeres but what about factors that can preserve or lengthen them? Stress, unhealthy weight, inactive lifestyles, and unhealthy diets are ways to shorten telomeres and speed up aging. Although scientists believe there are many factors to preserving telomeres, it appears diet plays the largest role.

With so much research around a vegan diet, studies have provided impressive data. For instance, a yearlong study was conducted with 400 women. The women were put into four groups. Each group consumed the same types of food like meat, grains, vegetables, and fruits. Telomere lengths were measured before the study and compared after the study. The first group was the control group and changed nothing about their daily lives. The second group consumed the same amount of food as the control group, but maintained weekly, vigorous exercise. The third group consumed the same diet as the control group but in lesser portions. And lastly, the fourth group maintained weekly, vigorous exercise like group two and the same diet but in lesser portions like group three. After a year, telomere lengths were measured again in all four groups. Astoundingly, there was little to no change for any group in telomere lengths. In conclusion, this study showed that it increasing exercise or limiting portion control does not affect telomere length as long as the same, lousy diet is being consumed (Mason, et al., 2013).

In a different, but similar study, a group of 30 men participated in a three-month study consuming only plant-based foods. The participants only endured light exercise, much different from the vigorous exercise being performed in the first study. When telomere lengths were measured after three months, a significant change in telomere length resulted. Telomeres were much longer then before the start of the study (Ornish, et al., 2008).

These studies show that exercise and weight loss did not directly affect telomeres, whereas the change in diet did. The study claimed that within a plant based diet the higher consumption of vegetables, less butter, and more fruit directly lead to the positive impact (Tiainen, et al., 2012). Furthermore the elevated consumption of foods high in vitamins and fiber also impacted the telomere health (Shalev, et al., 2013). The link between saturated fats, telomere length, and aging was also clear. Eliminating saturated fats from animals for just three months, was thought to be a heavy player in the significant outcome between the studies (Ford, 2010). From the studies, researchers were able to calculate the exact numbers of telomeres that would be affected by just eating one serving of ham or a hot dog.

Veganism for Ethical Reasons

Animal Cruelty (Warning: Sensitive Information)
In addition the health benefits received from the vegan lifestyle, deciding to go vegan is a great choice benefiting animals. As the world's population increases, the need to produce food at a high rate also increases. Many farmers feel the pressure to produce high quantity and quality sometimes gets put on the back burner. In order for many farmers to stay in business, more and more product needs to be produced to compete within the market.

For cattle, the cruelty starts at a young age. At a very young age cows are branded using hot metal irons, horns are cut or burned off, and male cows are castrated. Then, these animals are placed into tight, filthy living quarters. While being crammed together, cattle are fed an unnatural diet to fatten them up before being slaughtered. In addition, cattle are often given a dose of drugs to help them grow larger, quicker. Many cattle experience diseases due to the tight living quarters and additionally are fed with antibiotics. For female cows, they are often impregnated until they reach exhaustion to which then they are executed. While living, females are overexploited for their milk and are also given medications to increase milk production.

It's estimated that a cow's life expectancy is around 20 years, but many don't live past the age of five or six years before they are executed (Cruelty to Cows: How Cows Are Abused for Meat and Dairy Products: Animals Used for Food: Issues, n.d.). The bond between a calf and their mother is so strong that even though they are separated at birth by the meat industry, some will escape and travel great distances looking for their young. Sadly, many cows are thought to be conscious for a long period of time after the initial slaughter method (a shot to the head). Afterwards, additional slaughtering occurs until the cattle eventually dies. Pigs receive similar treatment and are confined to small spaces ridden with manure, diseases, insects, and dead animals.

Unlike vegetarians, many vegans are against the consumption of eggs due to the inhumane way they are produced. What many don't know is that chickens are intelligent animals and have intellect comparable to cats and dogs. Chickens, male or female, are jam packed into tight living quarters, many of which are filthy due to the amount of chickens living in the small space. Young chicks are separated from their moms and are raised initially in incubators along with many other chicks. In an egg farm, after being born females are sent to produce eggs right away.

Male chickens, as they do not produce eggs, are often dispelled inhumanely. Females promptly have their extremely sensitive beaks removed with a hot blade so they don't injure each other within their small cages. Due to the disease and illnesses associated with housing hundreds of chickens together, many are pumped with medications and some result in deformities as the chicken grows. Many chickens aren't able to stand up or lie down due to the amount of chickens living in one cage. Chickens normally prefer to stay clean but are unable to due to cages being stacked on top of each other. Waste falls from cage to cage, which is especially stressful considering naturally they are very hygienic animals. Chickens have a normal life span of 10-15 years, but usually only live about two miserable years in the egg industry. During slaughter, some chickens live until they are placed in boiling hot water used to remove their feathers. Other, fortunately, pass instantly when their necks are snapped after a miserable life.

Not only are animals treated horribly for food, many animals are also chemically tested on and killed for fashion items.

For the Environment
What many don't realize is the impact producing animal products takes on the environment. Supplying the whole world with meat and dairy products is not an easy task with over seven billion people to account for. Studies have shown that just one individual cutting down on their meat consumption can positively affect the environment. Research done by an Oxford University (2018) study showed that an individual eliminating meat and dairy products from their diet can reduce their personal carbon footprint by up to 73%.

Your carbon footprint is the stamp you leave on the Earth in regards to carbon emissions. What a person consumes, how much water and electricity is used day to day, recycling, and how sustainable someone is all contributes to a personal carbon footprint. If everyone eliminated or cut back on animal products, carbon footprints would drastically reduce as shown by the Oxford study (2018). In addition, the meat and dairy industry takes a toll on available land. The elimination of meat and dairy products would reduce total farmland use by 75% (Poore & Nemecek, 2018). This area is equivalent to the size of the US, China, Australian and EU combined (Petter, 2018).

This data shows how much land is being used to supply animal products when in reality, meat and dairy account for low amounts of calories and protein. It's important to take into account that not all of the world's population has access to meat and is considered more of a luxury item. With all of this being said, animal consumption uses a huge portion of land that could be used for other plant-based products. The lead author of the Oxford study, Joseph Poore (2018) explains, "A vegan diet is probably the single biggest way to reduce your impact on planet Earth, not just greenhouse gases, but global acidification, eutrophication, land use and water use."

The meat and dairy industry takes a heavy toll on water use. Many countries are experiencing a shortage of water or don't have a reliable water source. Water shortages can happen anywhere and don't have everything to do with poverty status. During an interview with the Guardian Sir James Bevan, chief executive of the Environment Agency warned that England could run short of water within just 25 years (Carrington, 2018). The meat industry uses tons of water to produce small amounts of food. For example, two pounds or nearly one kilogram of steak requires 4,800 gallons or over 18,000 liters of water (Skylark-Elizabeth, 2013). Yearly, those become unfathomable when considered the amount of steaks produced each year. One of the best ways to conserve water is to make the switch to a plant based diet. A plant-based diet used five times less water than a diet including meat (Vanham, Comero, Gawlik, & Bidoglio, 2018).

Pollution and Carbon Emissions
Deciding to partake in a vegan lifestyle can drastically reduce pollution and greenhouse gases. Scientists are in agreement that man affects the atmosphere of the earth made pollutants. The effects and outcomes may be disputed, however, scientists know that man-made pollutants are in fact harming the Earth. According to the Food and Agriculture Organization of the United Nations (2006), the livestock sector generates more greenhouse gas emissions than transportation. Forms of transportation include cars, cargo trucks, planes, trains, and ships. With approximately 7.7 billion people living on Earth in 2019, these figures are alarming (Current World Population, 2019).

With 7.7 billion people living today, more greenhouse gas emissions are produced by livestock than humans accessing transportation. A single cow can produce 70 to 120 kilograms of methane each year and there's an estimated 1.5 billion cows and bulls (Pradhan, et al., 2019). A Japanese study showed that a single car would have to drive 250 km (155 miles) to emit the same emissions as one kilogram (2.2 pounds) of beef (Ogino, Orito, Shimada, & Hirooka, 2007).

The problem with methane is that it's extremely potent. In turn, tons of methane is released into the atmosphere. A study by Princeton University (2014) revealed that methane is thirty times more potent than carbon dioxide, a widely known pollutant. Methane is considered a heat trapper. When the sun hits the earth, rays are absorbed by the land and atmosphere. Molecules from methane or carbon dioxide that are floating in the air absorb energy from the sun and readmit it. This process keeps the earth at a comfortable temperature where humans can live. When methane and carbon dioxide molecules rapidly increase from pollutants, more energy is absorbed and more heat is given off by the molecules. Methane is able to absorb much more energy than carbon dioxide making high levels much more dangerous. Pollutants like methane can lead to decreased life expectancy, trouble breathing (especially in elderly), asthma aggravation, low air quality, and smog.

Many have heard of climate change and global warming. Although both are controversial topics, science and data shows the direct effect high levels of methane and carbon dioxide have on the Earth. When methane escapes into the air, the molecules absorb the heat from the sun. The more molecules present in the air, the more the atmosphere gets warmed. This is the general basis for global warming. Global warming deals directly with greenhouse gases that are caused by humans and have documented the increase over the years.

Global warming changes the natural water cycle that deals with rainfall, evaporation, snow, stream flow and the melting of ice in the oceans. In turn temperatures, and sea levels rise causing a higher chance of natural disasters and flooding. Global warming also interrupts how agriculture normally grows because temperatures and the water cycle is affected. Higher temperatures and warmer water in normally cool regions is a problem because it interrupts the natural flow of the Earth. Heat related illnesses, cardiovascular problems, air quality issues, and lung issues all arise from global warming.

Chapter 2: All About Keto

The Ketogenic diet, Keto for short, has become increasingly popular over the years. The diet can be traced back to ancestral times to hunters and gathers many years ago. In the 1970's the Keto diet got a new start when it was implemented into epilepsy care and scientific research around the diet began. In today's world, the Keto diet is being used to treat obesity and is linked to the prevention and treatment of many other diseases. The Keto diet is a high fat, low carbohydrate diet. Protein also plays a role, but overall fat is the main player. When the body consumes high amounts of fats and little to no carbs, a new metabolic process occurs called Ketosis. Ketosis is a fat burning state and is the reason why the Keto diet has become so successful in weight loss. Ketosis is completely natural and arguably an overall better way for the body to function.

Keto 101

What is Ketosis?

Ketosis is a metabolic fat burning state in which the body burns fat for fuel. In a non-restrictive diet foods like bread, pasta, rice, cereals, and potatoes are consumed frequently. Grains, legumes, and starchy vegetables contain high amounts of simple carbs. The Keto diet restricts foods high in these simple carbs and replaces them with foods high in fat and complex carbohydrates. In turn, the body finds a new fuel source and Ketosis occurs.

Ketone bodies help regulate and maintain normal levels of hormones. Two major hormones that play a key role in appetite are Leptin and Ghrelin. Leptin is a hormone made by fat cells in the body's tissues. Leptin signals to the brain to stop eating and is considered a satiating hormone. When an individual has a high amount of body fat, Leptin levels are usually high as well. However, even though Leptin levels are high the individual may still endure cravings and the feeling of hunger. This is because like insulin, cells can develop a resistance to Leptin as well. Ghrelin is almost the opposite to Leptin. Ghrelin is a hormone created and released primarily in the stomach. This hormone lets the brain and body know that it's hungry and should consume food. When the body is in Ketosis, ghrelin is suppressed and cravings are put in check. A high fat diet allows ketones to keep the body full. Proper digestion and weight loss are among the benefits of lowered ghrelin.

When carbs are consumed and present in the body, Glucose is used for fuel. Glucose is a form of sugar made by the liver that supplies cells and organs with energy. At the same time, a hormone called insulin facilitates this process. Insulin allows the body to use glucose for energy by opening the barriers to the cells, similar to a key unlocking a door. Insulin is made in the pancreas and is responsible for regulating blood sugar levels. After glucose is produced by the liver the body signals the pancreas to produce insulin to facilitate. Together the two supply energy to the body and cells. After this process, a signal is released by the brain to the pancreas to shut off insulin production because the body is energized and has what it needs. In certain cases, this signal may become weak or muddied, and the pancreas continues to produce insulin because the signal to shut off production was not received.

Insulin is responsible for storing fat and sugar within the body. There are two reserve options for insulin to store unneeded sugar. The first is the sugar glycogen reserve, which can hold about 1,700 calories (Dolson, 2019). The second reserve is the fat reserve. When the small, sugar glycogen reserve is full insulin then stores sugar in the fat reserve, which leads to weight gain. Certain foods can be converted into sugar quicker, carbs being an example. Because carbs can be converted into sugar so easily this leads to quick, but unsustained energy. Blood sugar levels spike and high amounts of sugar are present. The body may not need all of this sugar thus leading to stored fat. High carb foods are known to have a high glycemic index while fats are considered to have a low glycemic index. Foods with a low glycemic index are preferable on the Keto diet because they provide low and sustained energy.

High sugar levels over a long period of time induce insulin resistance. Insulin resistance occurs when high amounts of sugar run through the body. High levels of sugar over a long period of time are toxic to the body so the body develops a resistance to protect the cells. In this situation, more and more insulin is produced because the body needs higher levels to respond and use the insulin. In addition, the communication between the brain and pancreas becomes blocked and the pancreas continues to produce large amounts of insulin. According to Dr. Eric Berg DC (2019), per one and a half gallon of blood, one teaspoon of sugar would represent a normal blood sugar level within the body. With that being said, the average American consumes 31 teaspoons daily (Berg, 2019). This amount equates to 140 pounds of consumed sugar, yearly. High blood sugar levels over time cause other health problems within the nervous system, eyes, heart, and brain so the body works hard to regulate these levels.

Replacing simple carbs with high fat and complex carbs, like those found in most fruits and vegetables, over time will lead to the body producing ketone bodies. Ketone bodies are a type of salt acid made by the liver when glucose is absent. Ketone bodies are only produced in the absence of carbs. Ketones are water-soluble molecules made of acetoacetate, beta-hydroxybutyrate, and acetone. Acetoacetate is formed first within the liver. When this chemical leaves the liver it then becomes beta-hydroxybutyrate. Beta-hydroxybutyrate is the most usable ketone and is the ketone that supplies the brain with energy.

Beta-hydroxybutyrate has an easy time entering the cell and is converted back into acetoacetate. The mitochondria of the cell then convert the ketone into energy that the body can use. When acetoacetate dies within the body, the third type of ketone is produced. Acetone is harmless in small amounts and is produced when the body doesn't convert acetoacetate into beta-hydroxybutyrate. In essence, when the body has enough energy, acetoacetate will dissolve itself before ever getting to the cells.

The Benefits of Ketones
Many scientists agree that Ketones are a great source of fuel for the body. The brain in particular, loves using ketones as a source of energy. This is due to better efficiency within the cells of the brain. Because Ketones have the capability to trigger a greater response within brain cells, many participants on the Keto diet experience increased cognitive functions. Mitochondria is considered the powerhouse of a cell and is responsible for taking in nutrients, breaking them down, and converting them into energy.

Ketones hold more energy per unit of oxygen than glucose, the source the brain usually utilized. Ketones also have the ability to create more mitochondria within the brain. This means that not only is more power utilized by cells, but more efficient cells are being produced at the same time. A study published in the journal of Molecular Brain Research (2004) found that ketones increase the amount of gene expression within mitochondrial enzymes in the brain. What this means is that genetic makeup changes, and better mitochondria production occurs leading to more energy, a feeling of calmness and a better ability to focus.

In addition, the Keto diet improves the ability to turn Glutamate into Gabba. Glutamate is a hormone within the brain that's responsible for the feeling of chaos, nervousness and anxiety. Gabba is the hormone that allows you to think clearly, and feel calm. Normally, the brain will convert extra glutamate into Gabba but someone with an unhealthy lifestyle will have a harder time with this process. This results in extra glutamate sitting stationary, causing stress and anxiety. A study by blank explained how ketones could aid in converting Glutamate into Gabba quicker and more efficiently than glucose (Lutas & Yellen, 2013). This means a better mood and enhanced clarity is more readily achievable, while still boasting tons of energy.

Tips for the Keto Diet

Keto Flu

The Keto Flu is a condition that brings flu type symptoms during the first stages of the Keto diet. Symptoms include dizziness, drowsiness, fatigue, constipation, muscle aches, nausea, insomnia and irritability. The good news is Keto Flu does not last long and can be avoided. Keto Flu is brought on when the body is adjusting to ketone bodies as a source of fuel rather than glucose. Glucose withdrawals are the main reason for some of these symptoms. While some experience Keto Flu, many do not. The severeness of Keto flu will depend on the participant's lifestyle beforehand. When starting a Keto-Vegan diet it's extremely important to stay hydrated. Consider adding a pinch of sodium like sea salt or Himalayan salt to water, and use a generous amount in meals. Drinking Keto friendly electrolytes is also recommended to help the body stay hydrated. Minerals like potassium and magnesium should be eaten in large quantities to help prevent Keto Flu.

MCT Oil

Medium Chain Triglycerides or MCT oil is made from a high concentration of coconut oil. MCT oil takes all of the nutritional benefits from coconut oil and condenses them into a stronger concentration. MCT oil contains a high amount of fats and unlike other fats is able to be digested quickly and used for energy. MCT oil is a great way to meet fat macros. MCT oil is completely natural and is good for brain health, cardiovascular health, neurological health and contains antibacterial components.

Soda

Although many sugar-free soda labels may seem harmless, there are many reasons why soda is not good for the body. Aspartame is a popular ingredient found in sodas that replaces traditional sugar. However, aspartame is inflammatory and irritates the lining of the stomach, which in turn triggers an unnecessary response from insulin. In addition to aspartame sodas contain unnatural ingredients and chemicals. Phosphoric acid is another example that causes tooth decay. If soda is a staple look for natural sodas or sparkling water that is sweetened by Stevia.

Food Apps

Especially in the beginning, a food app may be beneficial to track daily fat, protein, and carb intake. Documenting foods will help keep an individual on tract and aware of the calories being consumed as well. It's a great idea to get familiar with foods and what they contain to make the Keto-Vegan diet a smoother transition. Using a food scale may also be beneficial to measure out portions.

Exercise

Although exercise isn't completely necessary to lose weight while on the Keto-Vegan diet, it is recommended to stay active. Exercise brings many other benefits besides weight loss like stress prevention, better sleep, and the release of endorphins. Exercise has also been proven to help fight anxiety and depression. The best exercises while on the Keto-Vegan diet include low-intensity cardio, cycling, yoga, jogging, walking and swimming. Avoid exercises like HIIT, circuit training and intensive weight lifting, especially at the beginning.

Clear out the Kitchen

Choosing to start a new lifestyle is a challenge on it's own. Avoiding temptations and unhealthy foods are a lot easier when they aren't accessible. If possible, rid the pantries of old unhealthy snacks and replace them with new. The Keto-Vegan diet promotes healthy nutritious foods that are beneficial for those not on a Keto diet. Children and spouses will get used to the change and will receive great nutritional benefits as well. Another tip to prevent binging or unhealthy foods is to keep healthy snacks on hand. Nuts, seeds, and other Keto-Vegan snacks are great to carry in a purse, gym bag, car, or in a work desk. Having healthy snacks on hand will help reduce the urge to eat unhealthy snacks when hungry.

Chapter 3: What to Eat

When deciding what to eat on the Keto-Vegan diet, there are a few things to know. The keto diet is a macro-based diet which means specific macronutrients and micronutrients are looked at rather than calories. Macronutrients and micronutrients are certain compounds that the body needs. The difference between the two is macronutrients are needed in higher amounts and micronutrients are needed in small quantities. Depending on the weight loss plan, a small calorie deficit can be put in place, but know that the Keto diet is successful without severely restricting calories. This guide will go through the general macro and micronutrient needs but know that each person is a bit different. Our age, lifestyle, genes, or preexisting conditions all may slightly alter macro and micro nutrient counts.

Macronutrients

In regards to the Keto-Vegan diet the macronutrients are fat, protein, and carbs. The typical breakdown on a Keto diet requires daily intake of food to be 70% fats, 25% protein, and 5% carbs. These ratios may slightly change person to person depending on activeness, age, body composition or predetermined health problems.

Fats
There are four types of fats in a standard diet. It's important to know that not all fats are created equal. Although a Keto-Vegan diet requires a high amount of fats, there are certain fats to prioritize over others.

Monounsaturated fats, along with polyunsaturated fats, are the best types of fat to look for within food. Monounsaturated fats can be found in avocados, almonds, cashews, pumpkin seeds, peanut butter, chia seeds, olive oil, and sesame seeds. Monounsaturated fats can help reduce bad cholesterol levels, which in turn leads to a lower risk of heart disease and stroke. Monounsaturated also contain powerful compounds that work to maintain and promote the health of the body's cells. Many monounsaturated fats also are high in Vitamin E, which is a powerful antioxidant.

Polyunsaturated fat is another great fat to consume. Pine nuts, walnuts, Brazil nuts, flax seeds and sunflower seeds all contain amounts of polyunsaturated fats. Grapeseed oil also contains high amounts of polyunsaturated fats and is a great substitute for butter on a vegan diet. High amounts of omega-3 and omega-6 are found in polyunsaturated fats. Omega-3 cannot be produced by the body and can only be found in food sources. The Omega's are essential to the body and aren't found in many foods making many individuals deficient in this nutrient. Omega acids are important for brain development, brain function, blood pressure management, and heart health.

Saturated fats are by far the most common and widely known fats. Many studies around these fats have proven to be controversial in regards to their role on the body. The link between saturated fats and their influence on cholesterol is not clear causing some room for concern. In the past, cholesterol was indefinitely linked to heart disease. Recent studies have proven that this assumption is much more complex. Many of these studies dealt with saturated fats from animal products as saturated fats are mostly found in meat and dairy.

Coconut oil and cocoa are two examples of plant-based saturated fats and boast numerous health benefits. Coconut oil has properties that are antibacterial, and cancer fighting in addition to promoting brain health, skin health, and weight loss. Coconut oil is easy to cook with and other coconut products should be utilized while on a Keto-Vegan diet. Cocoa found in chocolate is also a saturated fat. Like coconut oil, cocoa contains a different type of saturated fat than animal products and is considered beneficial to the body.

The last type of fat, and the worst, is trans fat. There are no naturally occurring trans fats in vegan foods, which is good news. However, be sure to check the label of store bought food as trans fat is manufactured in food production.

Protein
Protein is essential to the body and cells. Cells need protein to build and repair tissues, make enzymes, hormones and other essential chemicals. Protein aids in the health of bones, muscles, cartilage, skin, and blood. Vegan foods containing protein include nutritional yeast, pepitas/pumpkin seeds, lupini beans, tofu, hemp seeds, almonds, sunflower seeds and macadamia nuts.

Carbs
The Keto diet severely restricts simple carbs. There is a small allowance of carbs while on the Keto diet, but these should be reserved for carbs naturally occurring in foods. Many foods contain a small amount of carbs and that's okay. Traditional pasta, bread,

crackers and grains should be replaced. Typically 20-30 grams of carbs is recommended to start with.

Micronutrients

Micronutrients are essential vitamins and minerals that are needed by the body. These vitamins and minerals can be divided into four categories: water-soluble vitamins, fat-soluble vitamins, macro minerals, and trace minerals.

Water-Soluble Vitamins

Water-soluble vitamins are simply vitamins that dissolve in water. The majority of vitamins are in this category. Because these vitamins are water-soluble, they dissolve and are flushed out of the body rather quickly. These vitamins are not able to be stored within the body for later use. Water-soluble vitamins play an important role in producing energy and triggering important chemical reactions within the body. Vitamin B is an example of water-soluble vitamins. Vitamin B1 can be classified as thiamine, B2 as riboflavin, B3 as niacin, B7 as biotin, and B9 as folate.Vitamin C or ascorbic acid is also an example of a water-soluble vitamin. Of these vitamins Vitamin B3, B7, B9, and Vitamin C have the highest recommended daily doses. Foods like leafy greens, avocados, almonds, spinach, and bell peppers will help reach most daily water-soluble vitamin goals.

A vegan diet can provide every vitamin needed except for one, and it falls into the water-soluble vitamin category. Vitamin B-12 is a vitamin that should be paid attention to while on the Keto-Vegan diet. Interestingly, the vegan diet is not the only diet low in B12. Individuals not participating in a vegan or vegetarian diet may still be deficient in B12. Years ago, this vitamin could be obtained from a plant based diet, but times have changed. Plants lose any B12 microbes they might have when they are washed because B12 organisms are stripped away. B12 is a microbe found in soil. B12 is essential for neurological function particularly within the brain. The reason why animal products contain B12 is because animals eat high amounts of soil. Individuals who do eat meat may still be deficient in B12 because many animals are not eating from high quality or nutrient dense soil.

B12 is a hard mineral to come across and animals are only able to receive it only because the amount of soil they eat is substantial. Jo Robinson (2013) from the New York Times explains, "Studies published within the past 15 years show that much of our produce is relatively low in phytonutrients, which are the compounds with the potential to reduce the risk of four of our modern scourges: cancer, cardiovascular disease, diabetes and dementia. The loss of these beneficial nutrients did not begin 50 or 100 years ago, as many assume. Unwittingly, we have been stripping phytonutrients from our diet since we stopped foraging for wild plants some 10,000 years ago and became farmers." When participating in a vegan diet, pay attention to B12 levels or monitor levels with a blood test performed by a physician. B12 levels can be replaced with supplements and nutritional yeast. Many plant milks are also fortified with B12 so staying efficient is easy.

Fat-soluble Vitamins

Fat-soluble vitamins, unlike water-soluble, are stored in the liver and fatty tissues for later use. Fat-soluble vitamins do not dissolve in water and are best absorbed when consumed alongside a source of fat. Vitamin A, Vitamin D, Vitamin E, and Vitamin K are examples of fat-soluble vitamins. These vitamins are imperative to vision, organ function, immune system health, bone growth, bone development, and blood clotting. Most fat-soluble vitamins are needed in higher amounts than water-soluble. Consuming spinach, plant milk, sunflower seeds, almonds, leafy greens, pumpkin, and sunlight are examples of how to reach daily fat-soluble goals.

Macrominerals

Macrominerals are typically needed in large amounts daily. Many macro minerals are recognizable. Examples being calcium, phosphorus, magnesium, sodium, chloride, potassium, and sulfur. These macro minerals are responsible for bones, teeth, muscles, blood vessel function, cell function/structure, producing enzymes, regulation blood pressure, hydration, and nerve transmission. As you can see, major minerals play a part in just about every body function.

Macro minerals can be found in leafy greens, broccoli, almonds, cashews, seaweed, salt, celery, garlic, onions, and Brussels sprouts. In addition, later in the guide you will see recommendations for Himalayan salt in numerous recipes. Himalayan salt contains trace major minerals like potassium, magnesium, and calcium. Himalayan salt also contains less sodium per teaspoon. Himalayan salt is a great alternative to make food better tasting while managing sodium levels and also contains beneficial minerals.

Trace Minerals

Although trace minerals are needed in smaller amounts than macro minerals, they still play an important part inside the human body. Iron, manganese, copper, zinc, iodine, fluoride, and selenium are examples of trace minerals. Trace minerals provide oxygen to muscles, assist in the creation of hormones, metabolism function, tissue formation, and thyroid regulation. The brain and nervous system also use trace minerals to carry out certain tasks. Trace minerals are found in spinach, pecans, peanuts, cashews, brazil nuts, and seaweed.

The Best Keto, Vegan Foods

Oils

Olive Oil

Olive oil is arguably one of the best things to consume daily. Olive oil is linked to numerous health benefits. Reduced inflammation, brain health, better cholesterol, improved skin, cellular health, and antibacterial benefits are all linked to olive oil consumption in addition to the prevention and management of rheumatoid arthritis, heart disease, cancers, and stroke prevention (Leech, 2018). When consuming olive oil look for claims like extra virgin and first, cold pressed. This ensures the highest quality of olives during production and protects the beneficial compounds. Olive oil is considered a monounsaturated fat, one of the best fats to consume on the Keto diet and in general. Olive oil is great for sauces, dips and dressings or for giving extra flavor to a dish. Some people even consume olive oil on its own, by the spoonful.

Coconut Oil

Coconut oil is unique in that it's a saturated fat. While most saturated fats come from an animal source, coconut oil is completely natural and contains great nutrition. Coconut oil is made from the meat of a coconut and contains high amounts of MCT. Coconut oil contains six times the amount of fat in comparison to olive oil. In addition, coconut oil is rapidly digested and quickly converted into energy. When shopping for oil look for claims like organic, pure, cold pressed and unrefined to ensure the best quality. Coconut oil has a relatively high smoke point in comparison to other oils making it a great option to cook with. Having a high smoke point is important and means that the composition of the oil will not change when exposed to high heat. Coconut oil has properties that can reduce and control appetite, manage cholesterol, promote brain health, increase fat burning, kill harmful microorganisms, improve skin, and promote dental health (Gunnars, 2018).

Macadamia Nut Oil

Although macadamia nut oil isn't very popular, it should be. Macadamia nut oil boasts healthy monounsaturated fats and has the perfect ratio of Omega 3 to Omega 6. The ratio of one to one in regards to the Omegas is the best possible ratio, and allows the body to absorb high amounts of the rare nutrient. Macadamia nut oil has a low smoke point but is great for sauces, dressings, and adding extra flavor to a dish. Macadamia nuts are known to lower the risk for heart disease, regulate blood pressure, protect the brain, fight and prevent certain cancers, and manage weight gain (Berry, 2019).

Oils to Avoid

Although there are many other oils boasting wonderful nutrients and properties, here are the oils to definitely avoid. With so many healthy options on the market avoid vegetable oil, soybean oil, canola oil, and corn oil. Although these oils may sound harmless, most are made unnaturally by extreme measures and are infused with chemicals. Many of these oils do not have a high tolerance for heat and change into cancer-causing compositions when exposed to high temperatures. Opt for an oil containing healthy fats and minerals.

Vegetables

Vegetables are important whether an individual is on a diet or not and can directly lead to how the body feels and functions. The best vegetables to consume on a Keto diet all entail high nutrient counts and low carbs. Typically vegetables above the ground are lower in carbs. Avoid vegetables such as potatoes, sweet potatoes, peas, corn and carrots as they contain higher amounts of sugars, starch, and carbs.

Green Vegetables

Broccoli is one of the best vegetables to consume as it is high in Vitamin C and K. Broccoli contains high amounts of fiber, which is important for the digestive system. Potassium is another mineral found in broccoli that is a great substitute for bananas since they are not Keto friendly. Broccoli is very versatile and can be used in soups, salads, casseroles or in a main dish. Broccoli contains nutrients that have the ability to decrease insulin resistance, a common barrier in weight loss and diabetes management.

Asparagus contains lots of vitamins while being low in carbs and calories. Vitamins A, C, E, K, potassium and folate are found in asparagus. Folate is especially vital for women in pregnancy because folate is known to aid in DNA development and cellular health. Small amounts of the rare mineral chromium is also found in asparagus and can reduce anxiety and depression symptoms.

Zucchini is a staple in a Keto-Vegan diet not only due to its nutrients, but for its versatility. Zucchini can easily be made into noodles using a spiralizer and is a great way to consume "pasta" dishes and lose weight. Zucchini is high in antioxidants and boosts heart and cardiovascular health.

Spinach and kale are two of the best lettuces to consume. Both are great for salads but can be added into other dishes as well. Spinach and kale contain lutein and zeaxanthin which are imperative to eye and retina health. Lutein and zeaxanthin work to protect the eyes from harmful rays and preserve eye vision. Other properties in spinach and kale act in anti-aging and anti-inflammatory capacities.

Although avocados are a fruit, many people treat them like a vegetable. Avocados are considered a superfood, meaning they contain some of the highest levels of overall nutrition per serving. For a vegan diet, avocados aid in the consumption of healthy fats. Avocados contain more potassium per serving than a banana, which is not widely known. Avocados also contain high amounts of vitamins K, C, B5, B6, E and folate. Avocados are loaded with fiber and are considered low carb. Avocados can be used in almost any dish and are a great addition to a smoothie.

Other green vegetables that are Keto friendly include celery, green beans, brussel sprouts, other lettuces, cucumbers, jalapeno peppers, green peppers, artichokes, and okra.

Other Vegetables
Red bell peppers are great for fighting the common cold and other illnesses. Containing 169% of daily-suggested vitamin C, red peppers have a powerful effect on businesses. Red bell peppers are arguably the food highest in vitamin C content. Red bell peppers also contain carotenoids which are another type of antioxidant and vitamin A.

Cauliflower is a staple on a Keto-Vegan diet because it can be made into just about anything. Cauliflower is also a great replacement for potatoes, which are not allowed on a Keto diet due to their high levels of sugar and carbs. Fortunately, cauliflower is high in vitamins and minerals like fiber, vitamin B and choline. Choline is used for learning and memory and is great for brain health. Cauliflower can be made into "mashed potatoes," pizza crust, and "rice."

Although many consider garlic a spice or herb, garlic actually belongs in the vegetable family. Fresh garlic can add a lot of flavor to many dishes and hold high nutritional value. Garlic is high in anti-inflammatory properties and is known to be powerful for fighting disease and illnesses.

One of the best ways to receive probiotics is through sauerkraut. Sauerkraut is essential fermented cabbage and contains living bacteria that serves as probiotics. Probiotics help the stomach to fight off any foreign bacteria the body isn't used to. A healthy gut helps foods to digest better and controls bloating, constipation, and gas. Having a healthy gut is important and will help the body feel better after meals. In addition, probiotics are great for the immune system and hormones. Sauerkraut can be purchased in the refrigerated sections of grocery stores or can be made at home.

Other vegetables that are accepted on the Keto diet are mushrooms, cabbage, onions, eggplant, tomatoes, and radishes.

Nuts

Nuts are great to add to dishes, or for snacking to reach fat macros. Nuts keep the body full and satisfied throughout the day. Not all nuts are suitable for a Keto diet due to their high carb count. Below are some of the best nuts to consume while on the Keto diet.

Pecans

Pecans are extremely high in fats but contain few carbs making them one of the best choices. Pecans are extremely nutritious and contain Omega-9. Omega-9 is able to kill fat cells, which aids in weight loss. In addition, Omega-9 plays a vital role in nerve health and helps the body transmit signals from the brain to the nerves.

Macadamia Nuts

Macadamia nuts are also great for a Keto diet due to their high fat count. Macadamia nuts contain flavonoids, which are essentially a type of antioxidant. Macadamia nuts hold the perfect ratio between Omega-3 and Omega-6. The ratio allows the body to absorb the maximum amount of nutrients possible. The ratio of one to one between Omega-3 and Omega-6 is quite rare among foods and is a special component to why macadamia nuts are so nutritious.

Brazil Nuts

Brazil nuts are another suitable nut to be consumed on a Keto diet. Brazil nuts contain magnesium, zinc, calcium, Vitamin E, and Vitamin B's. Selenium is another compound found in Brazil nuts. Selenium supports the immune system and act as an anti-inflammatory agent. Selenium also helps prevent and repair cellular damage.

Other Nuts

While there are many nuts on the market to choose, check the label to be sure the nut is low in carbs. Pistachios and cashews are examples of nuts that should be consumed less frequently or in smaller amounts due to their higher carb count. Other nuts that are low in carbs include walnuts, hazelnuts, pine nuts, almonds and peanuts. When purchasing nuts, be cautious of salted and unsalted as some nuts contain hidden high sodium. Raw nuts are always best and contain the highest nutrition.

Seeds

Many don't realize that seeds are one of the best foods out there in regards to nutrition. Many seeds are high in fats, vitamins, and minerals while staying relatively low calorie and low carb. Seeds can be snuck into almost any dish and make a great addition when used as toppings.

Flax Seeds

Flax seeds are arguably the most nutritious seed there is. Flax seeds are beneficial to heart health, brain health, weight loss, and digestion. Flax seeds are full of fiber which contributes to weight loss and proper digestion. Ligands are found in flax seeds and are known to regulate estrogen giving flax seeds extra benefit to women. Flax seeds must be ground to receive their nutrition.

Chia Seeds

Second to flax, chia seeds are the next healthiest seed. Chia seeds are similar to flax but contain fewer calories and more fiber making them excellent for weight loss. Like flax seeds, chia seeds contain selenium, iron, calcium, copper, potassium and Omega 3's. Chia seeds are tasteless, unlike flax seeds, and may be preferred in some dishes.

Sunflower Seeds

Sunflower seeds have the same texture and crunch as a nut, which makes them easy to consume on their own. Sunflower seeds contain an array of nutrients that promote heart health, immune health, eyesight, and are anti-inflammatory. Sunflower seeds are best consumed raw or should be purchased with little to no salt added to receive the most nutrients. Like nuts, sunflower seeds contain lots of fat and are helpful in reaching fat macro goals throughout the day.

Other Seeds

Other seeds like hemp seeds, pumpkin seeds or pepitas, safflower seeds, and sesame seeds are also a good option while on the Keto diet.

Chapter 4: Intermittent Fasting 101

Intermittent fasting is a helpful tool that can be utilized while on a Keto-Vegan diet. Intermittent fasting is simply a practice, and is a free way to receive extra health benefits. When an intermittent fasting practice is put to use, an individual experiences change at the cellular level. Because cells run through the body and are responsible for just about every function, having healthy and strong cells is extremely important.

Intermittent Fasting and the Amazing Concept of Autophagy

Intermittent fasting or IF for short isn't a diet, but rather a meal-timing plan. Meals are strategically planned and consumed at a specific times allowing a long period of time without food. Likewise, food is consumed within a certain time frame. Many participate in IF because of its success for weight loss. Intermittent fasting won't deplete muscle mass but will instead maintain pre existing muscle and promotes muscle growth, tone, and density.

Certain mental benefits also come along with IF because during an extended period of no food, the brain goes into survival mode. Although this may sound alarming, this mode is actually beneficial because it allows the brain to focus intensively on the task at hand. Ketone bodies are also produced during this time providing the body with a clean and sustainable fuel source, which the brain knows to preserve.

In addition to weight loss and better brain function, IF promotes autophagy which is the body's natural recycling process of old or damaged cells. Autophagy removes debris and is a form of internal cleaning through a recycling process. When autophagy occurs, cells are able to eat up old or damaged cells and use them to become stronger. Instead of throwing away these cells and disposing of them, the body gets creative and finds a way to use waste to its benefit. In turn this decreases the amount of waste the body needs to dispose of and leads to optimal cellular health. This process encourages anti-aging effects inside the body and out. Skin starts to look younger and fresher while organs are able to remain in good health.

Starting a fast is simple but there are some things to take into consideration. Before starting a fast, it's important to eat foods that are higher in fiber because fiber keeps the body feeling full and satisfied longer than other macros. Fibers controls hunger and will likely push back and stomach growling. A smaller amount of fats should also be consumed in addition to the fiber due to the fact that fats digest slower than other macros. Consider eating a high fiber vegetable with coconut oil over the top, for example.

The time spent in a fasting state is different for everyone and may change over time. A shorter fast will still lead to physical benefits, but a longer fast will lead to more autophagy benefits because the body as more time to perform autophagy functions. A 16 hour fast is a good place to start or work towards. This is known as 16-8 fasting. For example, at 8:00pm (20:00) consume a small meal and then withhold from food until 12:00pm or 12:30pm the following day. The times can also be adjusted and an individual may wish to start their fast earlier in the evening. A 16 hour fast leaves an eight hour window to consume food throughout the day. Because most of the fast is spent sleeping, the 16-8 method is a good place to start. Autophagy benefits don't begin until the 16 hour mark so any fast below 16 hours will not receive autophagy benefits. After 16 hours, the autophagy benefits exponentially increase as time goes by. Some individuals work their way up to 18 to 20 hours fasting.

In addition to the 16-8 IF method, there are some other methods to be aware of. Unlike the everyday 16-8 method, the 5-2 method allows 5 days of regular timed eating, and two days fasting. In addition, the two days spent fasting heavily restricts calories. This diet is also called the Fast Diet, popularized by British journalist Michael Mosley. Women are recommended to eat 500 calories and men 600 calories.

Another method referred to as Eat-Stop-Eat requires a 24-hour fast one or two days a week. To properly carry through with this technique, an individual consumes dinner and doesn't eat again until dinner the following day. Other participants chose breakfast-to-breakfast or lunch-to-lunch fasting. It's important to eat the same amount of food during the eating period, as if the fast never happened. This method of IF is very difficult and isn't suitable for everyone. The most popular method of IF is arguably the 16-8 method mentioned above.

During a fast, coffee, herbal teas and water with lemon, lime or citrus juice added can be consumed. Coffee should be consumed black with no added cream or sweeteners. Even Keto or Vegan sweeteners should not be consumed as they trigger an insulin response. The caffeine in coffee aids in weight loss during a fast and also keeps the body satisfied. A study published by the Journal Cell Cycle (2014) showed that the polyphenols in coffee encourages cells to undergo autophagy at a quicker rate. So not only is drinking coffee allowed, there may be additional benefits in doing so. Plain tea is also allowed during a fast but the same rules apply, no cream or sweeteners. Plain water should be consumed throughout a fast to keep the body hydrated. Be sure to consume any vitamins during an eating window, as some do have the ability to break a fast, and many are better taken with food.

When the fast is over, there are some tips on what to consume first. A healthy meal of fats and proteins is suggested. However, be aware that mixing fats and carbs after a fast may regress progress. Carbs have the ability to make the cells more receptive and trigger insulin levels. When carbs are consumed with fat, both carbs and fat have the ability to enter the cell. Fat by itself does not have the ability to enter a cell so it's important to not consume carbs right after a fast to preserve progress.

Exercising during a fast is extremely beneficial for weight loss and muscle tone. Although exercise during the food period is beneficial as well, the best results from a workout come while in a fasted state. Significantly more fat is burned while being in a fasted state in comparison to workout out during the eight-hour food window. Overall, the most fat can be burned during the very end of a fast, but this can be a difficult time to workout. Endurance and strength levels may be quite low. Working out in the morning, or in the middle of a fast, is still a good option especially for those adjusted to an IF lifestyle.

Common Myths About Intermittent Fasting

IF is generally safe but has received some scrutiny over the years by misinformed people. It's important to listen to your body and not to push yourself too hard when implementing IF. Although a form of IF is beneficial to almost everyone, gradually increasing time spent fasting is okay. It's also important to consult with a physician when preexisting conditions exist.

One of the main myths in regards to IF is that you'll lose muscle mass. However, a recent study compared subjects who were implementing IF and those who were not. During the study the participants consumed all of the same foods, with the only difference being intermittent fasting. The study published by the Journal of Translational Medicine proved that those who were using IF burned more fat and preserved/maintained more muscle (Moro, Marcolin, Battaglia, & Paoli, 2016).

Another common concern deals with the speed of the metabolism. The idea that the metabolism will slow down or thyroid production will be harmed while intermittent fasting is false. IF does not restrict calories, yet controls when food is consumed. The weight loss portion of IF is not from a calorie deficient. The weight loss and benefits come from the timing of when food is consumed and not. In regards to the thyroid, the thyroid produces hormones and chemicals as needed. So it's fair to say that the thyroid is less active at certain times only because certain levels or hormones/chemicals aren't needed. During an eating window, the thyroid production returns to normal, as it should to take care of the body's state of being.

Remember that IF is not starvation. Most IF methods still require the same amount of calories in comparison to someone not practicing IF. Obtaining vitamins and minerals through food is always important, so remember to eat a healthy Keto-Vegan diet during eating periods.

Chapter 5: Meal Plans

Meal Plan

Now that you have all the information on why the Keto-Vegan diet is so beneficial, it's time to put it into action! Using the information given above, recipes that are ketogenic and vegan have been created. Each recipe is 100% vegan despite some of the titles, and keto approved. Making moderations to favorite foods will help you be successful in making the Keto-Vegan diet a lifestyle.

You'll notice in the recipes that sugar is swapped for Stevia. Stevia is a natural sweetener made from the Stevia rebaudiana plant. The sweetener is calorie and carb free. Some studies have shown Stevia to have benefits of it's own but most benefits come from just eliminating sugar all together. Stevia is much, much sweetener than sugar. For reference, 1 cup of sugar (200 grams) only constitutes for 1 teaspoon (4 grams) of powdered Stevia. Keep this in mind when putting into recipes. For every recipe calling for Stevia, the level can be adjusted to preference. Other Keto-Vegan approved sweeteners include sucralose, erythritol, xylitol, and monk fruit sweetener. However, because Stevia is completely natural, it should be your first pick.

Another moderation to know is that basic flour can be swapped for almond flour, coconut flour, ground flax meal, and psyllium husk flour. The great thing about the Keto-Vegan diet is that breads, pizza, desserts, and more can still be enjoyed by using a Keto-Vegan flour. All four of the flours are nutrient dense and work great!

Butter is another basic ingredient needed in most recipes. Butter is not vegan and shouldn't be used. Luckily olive oil, avocado oil, and coconut oil make for great substitutes and give the same texture. Many vegan items can be store bought. A great example is vegan "mayonnaise." Just be sure to check labels for carb and sugar content.

Many of the snacks given also double as desserts. Throughout the day consider snacking on your favorite nuts. Nuts will help daily fat macro goals, don't need to be refrigerated, and will keep the body full. Make a few of the recipes in larger quantities so you have them throughout the month.

Lastly, many of the recipes have more than one serving or can be doubled. Consider repeating some of your favorites or getting creative with all the new information you know! Meal prepping on weekends can be extremely helpful for the workweek. Many of the recipes vary in how much time is needed so switch them up as needed. Remember to leave a review and please mention some of your favorite recipes!

The Menu

Breakfast Options:

1. Tofu Scramble
2. Avocado Toast (Bread Recipe)
3. Smoothie, Almond Vanilla
4. Cinnamon Roll Pancakes
5. English Muffin and Eggs (Bread Recipe)
6. Granola Bar
7. Blueberry Muffins
8. Breakfast Tacos
9. Toast (Homemade Jelly Recipe)
10. Overnight Oats
11. Smoothie, Strawberry
12. Bagel Recipe
13. Chocolate Pudding
14. Pumpkin Bread
15. Breakfast Burrito
16. Hash Brown Patties
17. Cereal

Lunch Options:

1. Veggie Burger Wraps
2. Turmeric & Cauliflower Soup
3. Fajitas (Tortilla Recipe)
4. Greek Salad (Vegan Feta Recipe)
5. Chili
6. Basil and Pesto Sandwich
7. Lunch Box (Hummus Recipe)
8. Cesar Salad
9. Sushi Salad
10. Egg Salad
11. Tomato Soup
12. Fajita Salad (Sour Cream Recipe)
13. Pasta Salad
14. Tuna Salad
15. Cabbage Soup
16. Spinach Salad with Dressing
17. Bagel Sandwich

Dinner Options:

1. Asian Power Bowl
2. Veggie Pizza

3. Creamy Vegetable Stir Fry
4. Spaghetti with Homemade Sauce
5. Portobello Burgers
6. Nachos
7. Carbonara with Bacon
8. Broccoli Cheddar Soup
9. Shepherd's Pie
10. Falafel
11. Grilled Portobello with Spinach
12. Buffalo Bites
13. Rice and Beans
14. Zucchini Tomato Bake
15. Kebab with Fries
16. Red Curry
17. Chicken Nuggets

Snack Options:

1. Salt and Vinegar Chips
2. Cinnamon Trail Mix
3. Fat Bomb, Pecan Dream
4. Chocolate Ice Cream
5. Almond Butter Cookies
6. Crackers
7. Nut Butter
8. Fat Bomb, Mint Chocolate Chip
9. Carrot Cake Bites
10. Candied Nuts
11. Zucchini Chips (Taco Seasoning Recipe)
12. Coconut Clusters
13. Almond Flour Blondies
14. Edible Cookie Dough
15. Brownies
16. Peanut Butter Bark

Recipes For Breakfast, Lunch, Dinner and Snacks

Day One, Breakfast

Tofu Scramble

Time: 15 minutes

Serving Size: 2 servings

Ingredients:

- 16 ounce/450 grams firm tofu (1 block)
- ½ cup/100 grams salsa
- 1 cup/80 grams mushrooms
- Small onion, chopped
- 2 tablespoons/30mL nutritional yeast
- 1 teaspoon/5 grams Himalayan salt
- ¼ teaspoon/1 gram turmeric powder
- ¼ teaspoon/1 gram onion powder
- 1 tablespoon/15mL olive oil
- 2 tablespoons/30mL almond milk
- Pepper to taste

Directions:

1. Heat olive oil over medium heat for one minute. Add the block of tofu.
2. Add the tofu into the pan using your hands or a kitchen utensil, crumbling the tofu into small pieces.
3. Cook for 3-4 minutes and stir until the water from the tofu is mostly gone.
4. Add in nutritional yeast, turmeric, salt, pepper, and onion powder and cook for an additional 5 minutes.
5. In a separate pan, sauté mushrooms and onions over medium heat.
6. Add mushrooms and onions into the same pan as tofu and stir in almond milk and salsa.
7. Stir for additional 30 seconds until well blended.

Day One, Lunch

Although some meal preparation is required for these delicious vegan veggie burgers, considering making them on a Sunday and saving additional burgers for lunches or quick meals throughout the week! Veggie burgers can be served alongside Keto bread with additional Keto approved toppings.

Veggie Burger Wraps

Time: 55 minutes

Serving Size: 3 servings

Ingredients:

- 1 tablespoon/15mL olive oil
- ½ cup/100 grams onion of choice, finely chopped
- 1 tablespoon/15 grams garlic, minced
- ½ cup/115 grams celery, finely chopped
- 8 ounces/230 grams mushrooms, finely chopped
- 10 ounces/285 grams riced cauliflower (one bag)
- 1 teaspoon/5 mL Worcestershire sauce
- ½ teaspoon/2 grams sea salt
- 1 teaspoon/4 grams smoked paprika
- ¼ cup/32 grams almond flour
- 1 tablespoon/15 grams chia seeds
- 2 tablespoons/30 grams ground flax seeds (flax egg)
- 6 tablespoons/90mL water
- Lettuce (from head or romaine strips)

Directions:

1. Mix ground flaxseed and water in a cup and refrigerate for 20 minutes.
2. Preheat oven to 400 degrees Fahrenheit or 205 degrees Celsius.
3. In a saucepan over medium heat, sauté celery, garlic, and onions. After a few minutes add in cauliflower and mushrooms. Cook for 12 minutes total or until no moisture is left in vegetables.
4. Add in salt, paprika, and Worcheshire sauce to the vegetable mixture. Then add flax egg, almond flour, and chia seeds.
5. Set mixture aside to cool.
6. Line two baking sheets with parchment paper.
7. Using hands, form the cooled mixture into six patties. Grease hands if needed, as the batter should be sticky. (If the dough is falling apart, add more ground flaxseed.)
8. Cook for 30 minutes or until the patties are golden brown. Allow cooling to firm patties. Store in airtight container in the refrigerator.
9. Place veggie burgers in lettuce wraps to enjoy.

Day One, Dinner

Although this recipe requires a little time, the preparation time only takes about five minutes. This is the perfect snack to meal prep on the weekends and save for throughout the week. The spices and vinegar are optional and can be adjusted to preference.

Asian Power Bowl

Time: 35 minutes

Serving Size: 2 servings

Ingredients:

- 10½ ounces/300 grams firm tofu, in bite sized pieces
- 1 tablespoons/15mL coconut aminos
- ½ teaspoon/2 grams garlic, minced
- ½ small green cabbage, roughly chopped into strips
- 1 teaspoon/5mL coconut oil
- 1 small green onion
- ¼ cup/ 60 grams cilantro, roughly chopped
- ½ medium avocado, peeled and pitted
- 1 cup/220 grams broccoli florets, steamed
- large handful of kale, steamed
- Himalayan salt and black pepper to preference

For the Sauce:
- 2 tablespoons/30 grams almond butter
- 1 tablespoon/15mL coconut aminos
- ½ tablespoon/8 grams apple cider vinegar
- 1 teaspoon/4 grams Sriracha sauce (optional)
- 2 tablespoons/30mL almond milk, unsweetened
- 1 teaspoon/4 grams powdered Stevia or to preference

Directions:

1. Preheat oven to 425 degrees Fahrenheit or 220 degrees Celsius. Line a baking sheet with parchment paper.
2. Press excess moisture out of the tofu by placing tofu in cheesecloth, a clean dishtowel, or paper towels. Set tofu into large bowl.
3. Add in 1 tablespoon (15mL) coconut aminos, minced garlic, Himalayan salt, and pepper. Allow the tofu to sit in the marinade.

4. Whisk together all sauce ingredients and set aside or into refrigerator until ready to be consumed. A blender can also be used for this step.
5. Place the marinated tofu on the lined baking sheet and bake the tofu for 15 minutes. After 15 minutes, remove tofu and flip. Bake the tofu an additional 15 minutes or until the tofu is brown and puffy.
6. Place the cabbage in a skillet over medium heat. Add coconut oil as needed to prevent burning. Add in green onion, cilantro, Himalayan salt, and pepper. Allow the vegetables to simmer and remove from heat when vegetables are golden brown and soft.
7. Split the cabbage mixture into two serving bowls (or more if doubling the recipe).
8. Add kale, broccoli, avocado, and sauce to the bowls. Add tofu to the top and serve with Himalayan salt and black pepper.

Day One, Snack

Although this recipe requires a little time, the preparation time only takes about five minutes. This is the perfect snack to meal prep on the weekends and saves for throughout the week. The spices and vinegar are optional and can be adjusted to preference.

Salt and Vinegar Chips

Time: 4 hours

Serving Size: 3 servings

Ingredients:

- 2 medium cucumbers
- 1 tablespoon/15mL avocado oil
- 2 teaspoons/10mL apple cider vinegar (optional)
- 1 tablespoon/4 grams rosemary or thyme (optional)
- Sea salt to taste

Directions:

9. Preheat oven to 175 degrees Fahrenheit or 80 degrees Celsius
10. Slice cumbers as thin as possible using a knife or mandoline slicer.
11. Remove access water from slices using paper towels or cheesecloth.
12. In a bowl, toss cucumbers with oil, vinegar, and spices of choice.
13. Place cucumber slices on parchment paper.
14. Bake for 3-4 hours or until crispy.
15. Allow cooling and store in airtight container.

Day Two, Breakfast

Below is the recipe for Keto, Vegan bread. This recipe will come in handy for many other meals. Although a bit of time is required, having bread throughout the week will make many meals quicker and simple. To complete this recipe, add half an avocado on top two slices of bread. Top with olive oil, balsamic vinegar and spice of choice. Sliced tomato or sauteed onions and mushrooms also make an excellent addition.

Avocado Toast- Bread Recipe 1

Time: 1 hour

Serving Size: 15 slices

Ingredients:

- 2½ cups/ 320 grams blanched almond flour
- ½ cup/64 grams coconut flour
- ⅓ cup/43 grams flax meal
- ⅓ cup/40 grams ground psyllium husk (if using cups, add additional 2 tablespoons)
- 1 tablespoon/10 grams baking powder
- Pinch of Himalayan salt
- 2 tablespoons/30mL avocado oil
- 2 teaspoon/10mL apple cider vinegar
- 2 cups/480mL lukewarm water

Directions:

1. Preheat oven to 400 degrees Fahrenheit or 200 degrees Celsius.
2. Line a loaf pan with greased parchment paper.
3. In a large bowl, add dry ingredients and mix well.
4. Slowly add in wet ingredients (order does not matter).
5. Mix well and then use hands to knead dough for an additional minute. If the dough is too sticky, add a pinch of psyllium husk. The dough should come together easily.
6. Set dough aside for 10 minutes.
7. Place dough into loaf pan and create a round top on the center of the dough. The dough should have a smooth surface.

8. Bake for 50-55 minutes. Place a toothpick in the center after baking. If the toothpick comes out clean, the bread is finished. If not, return the pan to the oven but cover with tinfoil to prevent burning.
9. Allow the break to cool completely before slicing. Store in refrigerator in an airtight container.

Day Two, Lunch

This recipe super quick and can be made in a pinch. Many of the spices are optional and can be based to taste. This is a low calorie and carb soup but is still quite comforting. This is a great recipe for weight loss and detoxing.

Turmeric & Cauliflower Soup

Time: 15 minutes

Serving Size: 6 servings

Ingredients:

- 1 large cauliflower head, sliced into pieces
- 1 large carrot, peeled and cut into chunks
- 1 thumb size piece of ginger, sliced into pieces
- 2 tablespoons/ 30 grams turmeric
- 1 teaspoon/5 grams black pepper
- 2 teaspoons/8 grams Himalayan salt
- 1 cup/237mL coconut milk
- 1 teaspoon/5 grams curry powder (optional)

Directions:

1. Fill a large pot with water and bring to a boil. Add cauliflower, carrots and ginger. Cook for 20 minutes over medium heat or until vegetables are soft.
2. Place vegetables and water into blender. Blend vegetables until smooth. Return contents to pot.
3. Gradually stir in salt, turmeric, pepper and coconut milk. Let soup simmer for an additional 5 minutes.
4. Garnish soup with additional coconut milk and herbs of choice.

Day Two, Dinner

The best part about a Keto-Vegan diet is that many comfort foods can still be enjoyed with some modifications. The toppings for this pizza should include favorite Keto approved veggies like onions, mushrooms, peppers, spinach and can even include a small amount of vegan, shredded cheese. Be sure to use low carb marinara sauce or make homemade.

Veggie Pizza

Time: 1 hour

Serving Size: 4 servings

Ingredients:

- 1½ pound/680 grams cauliflower, riced and drained
- 3 tablespoons/45 grams ground flax seeds
- ½ cup/64 grams almond flour
- Pinch of sea salt
- ½ teaspoon/3 grams oregano

Directions:

1. Preheat oven to 400 degrees Fahrenheit or 205 degrees Celsius. Line a large baking sheet with parchment paper.
2. Place cauliflower in thin, clean dishtowel. Squeeze out as much moisture as possible.
3. In a bowl, mix the cauliflower, flax, almond flour, salt, and oregano. Use hands and mix the dough thoroughly.
4. Place the dough onto the parchment paper and form a pizza crust. The thinner and flatter, the better.
5. Bake the crust for 35 minutes. After 35 minutes flip the crust and bake for an additional 10 minutes or until crust is golden brown.
6. Remove crust from oven and add pizza toppings.
7. Return to oven for 5 to 10 minutes.

Day Two, Snack

The best part about this recipe is that it can be stored and packed into a gym bag, purse or desk. Trail mix is the perfect snack to munch on throughout the day as the nuts provide excellent fats, calories, and protein. This recipe recommends Stevia but other Keto sweeteners are also acceptable. Add in vegan dark chocolate chips if desired.

Cinnamon Trail Mix

Time: 20 minutes

Serving Size: 12 servings

Ingredients:

- ½ cup/75 grams shelled hemp hearts
- ½ cup/75 grams raw pepitas
- ½ cup/65 grams raw almonds
- 1 cup/100 grams pecans
- ½ cup/50 grams walnuts
- ¼ cup/32 grams coconut oil, melted
- 1 tablespoon/15 grams ground cinnamon
- 1 teaspoon/5 grams sea salt
- 2 tablespoon/25 grams Stevia (optional)

Directions:

1. Preheat oven to 350 degrees Fahrenheit or 177 degrees Celsius. Line a large baking sheet with parchment paper.
2. If desired, chop or crumble nuts into smaller pieces.
3. Add nuts and dry ingredients into large bowl. Gradually stir in coconut oil.
4. Add mixture to baking sheet in an even layer.
5. Bake the mix for 13-15 minutes until nuts look golden.
6. Remove from oven and allow cooling. Store in airtight container in the refrigerator for freshness.

Day Three, Breakfast

This recipe is perfect for quick mornings and can be taken on the go. Although this recipe plays to vanilla lovers, simply adding a bit of cocoa will make this recipe into a chocolate treat as well. The avocado makes this smoothie feel more like dessert giving it a creamy, delectable texture.

Protein Smoothie- Vanilla Almond

Time: 5 minutes

Serving Size: 1 smoothie

Ingredients:

- ½ avocado
- 2 tablespoons/30 grams almond butter
- 1½ cup/355mL almond milk
- 1 tablespoon/15mL coconut oil, melted
- 1 tablespoon/15 grams cocoa powder, unsweetened (optional)
- 1 teaspoon/5mL vanilla extract
- Pinch of sea salt
- Pinch of Stevia (optional)
- Handful of ice or to preference

Directions:

1. In a high-speed blender, add all the ingredients. Blend until smooth and well mixed.

Day Three, Lunch

Below is the recipe for Keto-Vegan tortillas. For today's lunch, consider sauteing peppers, onions, and mushrooms. Top with avocado, lettuce, tomato and vegan cheese. For a sour cream substitute, look for unsweetened, plant-based yogurts.

Tortilla Recipe- Fajitas

Time: 15 minutes

Serving Size: 4 tortillas

Ingredients:

- 1 cup/128 grams almond flour
- 3 tablespoons/25 grams ground psyllium husk
- ½ tablespoon/7 mL avocado oil
- ½ cup/125mL lukewarm water
- Pinch of onion or garlic powder (optional)
- Pinch of Himalayan salt

Directions:

1. In a bowl, stir together almond flour, psyllium husk, salt, and spices.
2. Gradually add avocado oil and water. Using a spatula, stir the mixture well. Then use hands to knead dough into a ball.
3. Separate the dough into four even pieces.
4. Place one of the pieces in between two pieces of parchment paper and press until a round tortilla forms. The thickness should be thin, but not falling apart.
5. On a non-stick or lightly oiled pan, cook tortilla over medium heat for 2-3 minutes.
6. Flip tortilla and cook for an additional 1-2 minutes. The longer the tortilla is cooked, the crispier it will become so be sure the center of the tortilla always remains soft while cooking
7. Store tortillas in plastic wrap in the refrigerator after cooled.

Day Three, Dinner

Creamy Vegetable Stir Fry

Time: 30 minutes

Serving Size: 2 servings

Ingredients:

- 1 cup/220 grams firm tofu
- 1 small onion, chopped
- 1 small red bell pepper, thinly sliced
- 1 cup/220 grams broccoli
- 2 cups/440 grams spinach, chopped
- 2 teaspoons/10mL coconut oil
- 2 tablespoon/30mL coconut aminos
- ½ cup/125mLwater
- 1 teaspoon/5mL sesame oil
- 3 ½ tablespoons/53 grams almond butter
- 1 teaspoon/4 grams garlic
- Salt and pepper to taste

Directions:

1. In a large pan sauté tofu, onion, red bell peppers, broccoli, and spinach using coconut oil over medium heat.
2. In a bowl, whisk together coconut aminos, water, sesame oil, garlic, salt and pepper.
3. When the vegetables are finished, pour in the sauce.
4. Add the almond butter and stir until melted and evenly mixed.

Day Three, Snack

Fat bombs are a great way to reach daily macro goals because they are high in healthy fats. Fats bombs are also extremely delicious and will definitely satisfy a sweet tooth.

Fat Bomb- Pecan Dream

Time: 1 hour

Serving Size: 18 fat bombs

Ingredients:

- ½ cup/63 grams pecans, ground
- ½ cup/118mL coconut oil, melted
- 18 whole pecans
- 1 teaspoon/5mL vanilla extract
- 1 tablespoon/8 grams stevia
- Pinch of sea salt

Directions:

1. In a large bowl, combine all ingredients excluding 18 whole pecans.
2. Place mixture into ice cube tray or mini cupcake liners. About two spoonfuls should go into making one fat bomb.
3. Freeze for 15 minutes.
4. Remove fat bombs from freezer and place one whole pecan atop each fat bomb.
5. Freeze and store in fridge.

Day Four, Breakfast

This is a Keto-Vegan take on cinnamon rolls. This recipe is sure to be loved by all but if cinnamon isn't a favorite, substitute with unsweetened cocoa powder and top with vegan, Stevia sweetened chocolate chips.

Cinnamon Roll Pancakes

Time: 20 minutes

Serving Size: 3 servings

Ingredients:

For the Pancakes
- 1 cup/90 grams rolled oats
- ½ cup/125mL almond milk
- 2 tablespoons/30 grams ground flax seeds (flax egg)
- 6 tablespoons/90mL water
- 1 tablespoon/15mL apple cider vinegar
- 1 teaspoon/4 grams baking powder
- 1 teaspoon/5 grams cinnamon (optional)
- 1 teaspoon/5 mL vanilla extract

For the Sauce
- 2 cups/160 grams coconut flakes, unsweetened
- 1/2 tablespoon/7mL coconut oil, melted
- 1 teaspoon/5mL cinnamon
- 1 tablespoon/15mL coconut milk

Directions:

1. Mix ground flaxseed and water and refrigerate for 20 minutes.
2. Place all ingredients in blender and blend until a thick batter forms.
3. Let the batter rest for 20 minutes until the flax egg is ready.
4. Mix in flax egg with spatula.
5. In ¼ cup increments, pour batter into a non-stick saucepan over low heat.
6. Cook until edges are firm and flip the pancake. Cook until both sides are golden brown.
7. Continue until no batter remains.

8. For the sauce, rinse the blender and add ingredients. Blend for 1 minute and pour on top of pancakes as desired.

Day Four, Lunch

This recipe only takes about 5 minutes to prepare and is a great addition to salads or meals throughout the week. For today's lunch, prepare a few favorite veggies and toss them over a salad along with feta cheese. Top off the salad with olive oil for dressing.

Greek Salad- Vegan Cheese Recipe

Time: 2 hours

Serving Size: 4 servings

Ingredients:

- 9.7 ounces/275 grams firm tofu
- ¼ cup/60mL lemon juice
- ½ cup/125mL water
- ½ cup/125mL apple cider vinegar
- 1 tablespoon/15 grams oregano
- 2 teaspoon/9 grams dried rosemary (optional)
- Salt and pepper to taste

Directions:

1. Press excess tofu from water using paper towels.
2. Cut the tofu into small cubes.
3. In a bowl, mix the lemon juice, water, apple cider vinegar, and spices.
4. Add the tofu pieces to the marinade bowl and cover. Refrigerate for two hours to allow the marinade to sink it.

Day Four, Dinner

This recipe is a Vegan-Keto approved recipe that is a take on traditional spaghetti. Regular noodles are not allowed in Keto so consider investing in a vegetable spiralizer. Zucchini is a great vegetable to turn into noodles, as they resemble a similar taste and texture to regular noodles. Keep in mind that store-bought marinara sauce may be hiding sugar and carbs so it's best to check the label or make homemade!

Spaghetti with Homemade Sauce

Time: 25 minutes

Serving Size: 3 servings

Ingredients:

- 2 medium sized zucchini
- 1 can crushed tomatoes
- 3 tablespoons/45mL olive oil
- 1 medium onion, chopped
- 1 garlic clove, chopped
- 1 cup/80 grams mushrooms
- Handful of spinach (lettuce form)
- 1 teaspoon/5 grams oregano (substitute or ass thyme, basil, or Italian herbs to preference)
- Pinch of red pepper flakes (optional)
- Sea salt and pepper to taste

Directions:

1. Using a spiralizer, form zucchini noodles. If a spiralizer is not owned, chop the zucchini into thin, round pieces. Set the noodles aside.
2. In a large pan, sauté onions over medium heat for 5 minutes or until soft.
3. Add chopped garlic, tomatoes, and spices.
4. Add in mushrooms.
5. Allow the sauce to simmer for 15 minutes.
6. Add the zucchini noodles into the mixture and cook for 3-4 minutes until the zucchini noodles are soft, but not soggy.
7. Add in a handful of fresh spinach.

Day Four, Snack

Ice cream can always be enjoyed on a Keto-Vegan diet! Although this recipe takes a bit of time in the freezer, the prep time is less than five minutes! Additional toppings can include macadamia nuts, pecans, peanuts, almonds, or a handful of berries!

Chocolate Ice Cream

Time: 2 hours

Serving Size: 4 servings

Ingredients:

- 3 large avocados, peeled and pitted
- 1 can/15 ounce full-fat coconut milk (445mL)
- 1 cup/118 grams cocoa powder
- 2 tablespoons/20 grams Stevia
- 1 teaspoon/5mL vanilla extract
- 1 teaspoon/5mL almond extract
- Pinch of sea salt
- ½ cup/90 grams vegan, stevia sweetened chocolate chips (optional)

Directions:

1. Place all ingredients except chocolate chips into a blender and blend until smooth.
2. Transfer contents into sealable container and freeze for 2 hours. When ready to eat, remove ice cream and let it thaw for a few minutes.

Day Five, Breakfast

This breakfast is simple, quick, and satisfying. Consider serving with tomato, onions, mushrooms, or avocado to make this breakfast truly gourmet.

English Muffin and Eggs

Time: 10 minutes

Serving Size: 1 serving

Ingredients:

For the Muffin:
- 1 tablespoon/15mL coconut oil, melted
- 1 tablespoon/ 7 grams ground flax seed
- 3 tablespoons/45mL water
- 3 tablespoons/25 grams blanched almond flour
- ½ tablespoon/5 grams coconut flour
- Pinch of Himalayan salt
- ½ teaspoon/2 grams baking powder

For the Eggs:
- 4 ounces/110 grams extra firm tofu
- ½ tablespoon/7mL olive oil
- 1 tablespoon/7 grams nutritional yeast
- ½ tablespoon/3.5 grams onion powder
- ¼ teaspoon/1.4 grams turmeric
- 3 tablespoons/45 mL almond milk
- Salt and black pepper to preference

Directions:

1. Mix the ground flax seed and water and place in refrigerator.
2. In a large pan, mash tofu-using spatula. Sauté in olive oil.
3. Add nutritional yeast, turmeric, onion powder, salt, and pepper.
4. Slowly add in almond milk and stir.
5. Cook tofu until desired consistency is reached.
6. In a ramekin or microwave safe mug, place almond flour, coconut flour, salt, and baking powder. Stir.
7. Remove flax egg from refrigerator and whisk into mug. Add melted coconut oil.

8. Microwave for 1 minute and then in 30 second increments until firm. This process should take less than two or three minutes.
9. Remove from microwave and serve with eggs.

Day Five, Lunch

This low carb chili is fantastic for a cozy afternoon. Consider topping with avocados, cilantro, keto tortilla chips, or vegan sour cream.

Chili

Time: 35 minutes

Serving Size: 6 servings

Ingredients:

- 1 tablespoons/30mL olive oil
- 3 stalks of celery, diced
- 1 medium onion, chopped
- 1 cup mushrooms
- 1 garlic clove, separated and chopped
- 1 teaspoon/4 grams ground cinnamon
- 1 teaspoon/4 grams chili powder
- 2 teaspoon/14 grams ground cumin
- 1 green bell pepper, diced
- 1 zucchini, diced
- 1 can diced tomato
- 1 cup/ water
- ¼ cup/63mL coconut milk
- ½ cup/63 grams raw walnuts
- ½ tablespoon/5 grams cocoa powder, unsweetened
- Salt and pepper

Directions:

1. In a large saucepan, sauté celery, bell peppers, zucchini, mushrooms, and onion in olive oil over medium heat.

2. Add in spices, diced tomatoes, water, coconut milk, and walnuts.
3. Simmer for 20-25 minutes or until vegetables are soft.

Day Five, Dinner

Burgers don't have to be a thing of the past while on a Keto-Vegan diet. In fact, these portobello burgers rival any other burger with their tastiness. The recipe for the burger is below. Top burgers with avocado, tomato, onion, and any other favorite toppings in between a Keto English muffin.

Portobello Burgers

Time: 30 minutes

Serving Size: 2 burgers

Ingredients:

- 2 medium or large Portobello mushroom caps
- 1½ tablespoon/ 23mL avocado oil
- 1 tablespoon/15mL balsamic vinegar
- ½ tablespoon/3 grams Italian seasoning
- 1 tablespoon/6 grams minced garlic
- Salt and pepper to preference

Directions:

1. In a bowl, mix all ingredients excluding mushrooms. Mix well.
2. Place mushrooms in marinade and place in the refrigerator for 10-25 minutes.
3. In a large saucepan, place mushroom caps face up. Cook for 5 minutes.
4. Flip mushrooms and cook for an additional 4 minutes. Remove mushrooms from heat when they appear golden brown.

Day Five, Snack

Almond Butter Cookies

Time: 15 minutes

Serving Size: 12 cookies

Ingredients:

- 1 cup/237 mL almond butter
- 1 tablespoon/10 grams Stevia
- 4 tablespoons/60 grams ground chia seeds
- 2 tablespoons/30 grams vegan, Stevia sweetened chocolate chips

Directions:

1. Preheat oven to 350 degrees Fahrenheit or 180 degrees Celsius. Line a large cookie sheet with parchment paper.
2. In a large bowl, mix almond butter, stevia, and ground chia seeds. The batter should be thick. Fold and gently mix in chocolate chips.
3. Form the dough into small balls and place on parchment paper. Recipe yields about 12 cookies.
4. Bake cookies for 10-12 minutes or until edges are golden.
5. Remove tray and allow cooking.

Day Six, Breakfast

Granola bars don't have to be a think of the past while on a Keto-Vegan diet. These granola bars pack tons of nutrients, healthy fats, and protein to jumpstart the morning. If chocolate is a favorite, another simple step can be added. Melt Stevia sweetened, vegan chocolate and dip the bottom of the bars after they have cooled down. Freeze the bars on parchment paper until the chocolate is solid.

Granola Bars

Time: 35 minutes

Serving Size: 8 granola bars

Ingredients:

- 2 tablespoons/14 grams ground flax seeds
- 2 tablespoons/22 grams chia seeds
- ½ cup/125 mL warm water
- 1 teaspoon/5mL vanilla extract
- ½ teaspoon/3 grams stevia powder
- ½ cup/60 grams pecans, crushed
- 2 tablespoons/30 mL almond butter, melted
- 1 tablespoon/15 mL coconut oil, melted
- 2 teaspoons/14 grams cinnamon
- ½ cup/80 grams hulled hemp seeds
- ¼ cup/25 grams shredded coconut, unsweetened
- 1 tablespoon/9 grams sesame seeds

Directions:

1. Preheat oven to 350 degrees Fahrenheit or 177 degrees Celsius. Line a large baking pan with parchment paper.
2. In a large bowl, mix flax, chia seeds, water, stevia, and vanilla. Stir well and set aside for 5 minutes.
3. Stir in almond butter, coconut oil, pecans, shredded coconut, hemp seeds, sesame seeds, and cinnamon.
4. Spread the mixture evenly onto the baking sheet. Smooth the top and edge the corners so a large rectangle is formed from the mixture.
5. Bake for 25 to 30 minutes or until edges turn golden brown.
6. Allowing cooling and slice into bars. Recipe should yield around eight. Store in airtight container in the refrigerator.

Day Six, Lunch

Basil and Pesto Sandwich

Time: 10 minutes

Serving Size: 1 serving

Ingredients:

- Keto-Vegan English muffin (See Recipe for Day 5, Breakfast)
- 1 small tomato, sliced
- Half avocado, peeled and pitted

For the Sauce
- 1 cup/24 grams basil leaves
- 3 tablespoons/40 grams sunflower seeds, raw
- 1 teaspoon/4 grams garlic, minced
- 2 teaspoons/10mL of olive oil
- 2 teaspoons/8 grams oregano
- Squeeze of lemon juice
- Himalayan salt and pepper to preference

Directions:

1. Add all the sauce ingredients to a food processor or blender. Add water as needed to create a smooth, but thick consistency.
2. Prepare English muffin using recipe from Day 5, Breakfast. Allow a brief cooling and slice the muffin in half.
3. Spread the sauce evenly on both slices of bread. Top sandwich with tomato and avocado.

Day Six, Dinner

This recipe is perfect for parties, weekends, or special occasions. Also perfect for game day, this recipe is sure to be loved by the whole household. These nachos can be topped with any favorite Keto-Vegan toppings such as lettuce, tomato, jalapeno peppers, and onions. Although this recipe takes a little time, cheese or meat can be omitted to speed up the process if necessary.

Nachos

Time: 45 minutes

Serving Size: 2-3 servings

Ingredients:

For the Chips
- 1 tablespoon/14 grams of chia seeds
- ¼ cup/60mL water
- 1 cup/128 grams blanched almond meal
- 1 tablespoon/15mL avocado oil
- 1 teaspoon/4 grams nutritional yeast
- Pinch of Himalayan salt

For the Cheese
- 1 cup/240mL macadamia nuts (soaked overnight if possible)
- 1 red pepper, sliced with no seeds
- 1 tablespoon/15mL olive oil
- 3 tablespoons/45 grams nutritional yeast
- 1 teaspoon/4 grams lemon juice
- ½ cup /130mL vegetable stock, low sodium
- ¼ teaspoon/1.5 grams onion powder

For the Meat
- 2 cups/450 grams raw walnuts
- 2 teaspoons/8 grams garlic, minced
- Small onion, chopped
- 2 tablespoons/30mL olive oil
- 2 tablespoons/8 grams nutritional yeast
- 2 teaspoons/8 grams ground cumin
- 1 teaspoon/4 grams cayenne pepper (optional)

- Himalayan salt and black pepper to preference

Directions:

Preparation
1. Place macadamia nuts in a bowl. Cover with boiling water. Cover the bowl and set aside. Best if soaked overnight.
2. Place walnuts in separate bowl. Pour cool water over the top. Set aside.
3. Preheat oven to 390 degrees Fahrenheit or 200 degrees Celsius. Line a baking sheet with parchment paper.

For the Chips
4. In a bowl, add chia seeds and water. Whisk or stir well. Set aside for 10 minutes.
5. In a different bowl, add blanched almond meal, olive oil, spices and the chia seed mixture.
6. Using hands, knead the mixture for about one minute.
7. Separate dough into three even pieces.
8. Roll a piece of dough into a ball and place the dough in between two pieces of parchment paper. Use a rolling pin to roll the dough as thin as possible.
9. Using a pizza cutter or knife, cut into the dough to create a triangle shaped chips. Place on lined baking sheet. Each piece of dough should yield 10 chips, 30 in total.
10. Bake the chips for six or seven minutes or until they appear golden brown. Keep in mind these chips have the ability to burn and should be checked on frequently after five minutes of baking.
11. Remove from oven and allow cooling. Use a flat tool to remove the chips from the parchment paper once cooled.

For the Meat:
12. Drain water from walnuts and add to food processor or blender. Add all other meat ingredients. Pulse until a ground meat texture is achieved.
13. Sauté onion and add to meat mixture.

For the Sauce:
14. In a skillet, sauté red pepper until golden brown.
15. Drain and rinse macadamia nuts.
16. Place red pepper, macadamia nuts, and remaining ingredients in blender. Blend sauce until smooth but no more than 30 seconds to 1 minute.

Day Six, Snack

This recipe is wonderful on its own or with a favorite Keto-Vegan dip. For a sweet snack, pair with a nut butter.

Crackers

Time: 1 hour, 15 minutes

Serving Size: 10 serving

Ingredients:

- 1 cup/125 grams sunflower seeds, raw
- ¾ cup/95 grams pumpkin seeds
- ½ cup/60 grams chia seeds
- ½ cup/65 grams sesame seeds
- ¼ cup/30 grams flaxseed
- 1½ cup/120mL water
- 2 tablespoons/25 grams thyme or rosemary
- Pinch of salt

Directions:

1. Preheat oven to 340 degrees Fahrenheit or 170 degrees Celsius. Line two baking sheets with parchment paper.
2. Mix all ingredients together and set aside for 10 minutes.
3. Stir mixture again and pour over lined baking sheets. Spread evenly. The crackers shouldn't be too thin or too thick.
4. Bake for one hour or until golden brown and crisp.
5. Remove from the oven and allow cooling. Break into chips.
6. Store in an airtight container.

Day Seven, Breakfast

Blueberry Muffins

Time: 25 minutes

Serving Size: 12 serving

Ingredients:

- 1¾ cup/224 grams blanched almond flour
- 2 tablespoons/25 grams Stevia
- ½ cup/64 grams tapioca flour
- 2 teaspoons/8 grams baking powder
- 4 tablespoons/60mL coconut oil
- ½ cup/125mL almond milk
- ½ cup/63 grams blueberries

Directions:

1. Preheat oven to 350 degrees Fahrenheit or 175 degrees Celsius. Lightly grease 12 count muffin tins. Set aside.
2. In a bowl add almond flour, stevia, tapioca flour, and baking powder. Mix well.
3. In a separate bowl mix together coconut oil and milk.
4. Add mixtures together and stir gently. Lightly add in blueberries.
5. Leave mixture to rest for 5 minutes.
6. Pour batter into muffin tins. Each tin should be about ⅔ way full.
7. Bake for 20-25 minutes until a toothpick comes out clean.
8. Transfer muffins onto counter for cooling.

Day Seven, Lunch

Today's lunch is similar to snack boxes bought at Starbucks or in a store. The lunch is super quick to prepare and contains great protein and fats. Below is a hummus recipe to accompany either Keto tortilla chips or crackers. In addition, slice cucumbers or peppers to accompany the hummus. Include a handful of berries and a handful of nuts.

Lunch Box- Hummus Recipe

Time: 5 minutes

Serving Size: 3 servings

Ingredients:

- 2 avocados, peeled and pitted
- ¼ cup/32 grams tahini
- ¼ cup/60mL olive oil
- ¼ cup/60mL lime juice
- ½ teaspoon/2 grams cumin
- Salt and pepper to taste

Directions:

1. Place all ingredients in a blender excluding olive oil. Pulse until the ingredients are well mixed and the desired texture is achieved.
2. Scoop mixture into a bowl and drizzle olive oil over the top.
3. Pack remaining items into lunch box (listed in description).

Day Seven, Dinner

This dish is the perfect recipe for a cozy night. This recipe calls for shirataki noodles, which essentially contain zero calories and carbs. The noodles are also fibrous adding additional benefit. If desired, zucchini noodles or any other Keto noodles could be swapped.

Carbonara with Bacon

Time: 40 minutes

Serving Size: 2 serving

Ingredients:

For the Tofu Bacon
- ½ block firm tofu (7oz/200g)
- 1 ½ tablespoons/23 mL tamari, low sodium
- 1 tablespoons/15mL avocado oil
- Pinch of smoked paprika (optional)
- Pinch of sea salt

For the Sauce
- ½ cup/80 grams hulled hemp seeds
- 2 tablespoons/30 grams nutritional yeast
- ⅓ cup/80 mL water
- 1 tablespoon/15mL avocado oil

For the Dish
- 1 package shirataki noodles (8oz/226 grams)
- 1 teaspoon/4 grams nutritional yeast
- 1 scallion stalk, sliced thin
- Sea salt and black pepper to preference

Directions:

For the Tofu Bacon
1. Preheat oven to 375 degrees Fahrenheit or 190 degrees Celsius. Line a baking sheet with parchment paper.
2. Drain the tofu and press lightly with a clean dishtowel or paper towels. Slice tofu as thin as possible. Around 12 slices total should be cut.

3. In a bowl, mix together tamari, avocado oil, salt, and smoked paprika.
4. Dip each piece of tofu into the marinade and lay onto lined baking sheet.
5. Pour an extra marinade over tofu and bake for 30 minutes or until crispy.

For the Sauce
6. Add all ingredients into a blender and blend until well mixed and smooth. This process should take two or three minutes to achieve the optimal texture.

For the Dish
7. Drain and rinse shirataki noodles. Place them in pan on low heat.
8. Add the sauce into the pan and stir.
9. Let the noodles and sauce simmer for 10 minutes. The sauce should thicken during this time.
10. When tofu bacon is complete remove from oven and chop into pieces. Stir the pieces into the pan. Simmer for two or three minutes.
11. Serve with nutritional yeast, scallions, salt and pepper sprinkled over the top.

Day Seven, Snack

Below is the recipe and directions to make nut butter. This recipe can be made with pecans, cashews, macadamia nuts, or walnuts as well. Nut butter can be eaten with crackers, celery, or on Keto toast.

Nut Butter Recipe

Time: 30 minutes

Serving Size: 4 servings

Ingredients:

- 2 cups/250 grams raw almonds
- 1 teaspoon/4 grams cinnamon (optional)
- ¼ cup/32 grams ground coconut (optional)
- Pinch of Himalayan salt
- Coconut oil, as needed (melted)

Directions:

1. Preheat oven to 325 degrees Fahrenheit or 165 degrees Celsius.
2. Place nuts evenly on unlined baking sheet and bake for 10 to 15 minutes. Stir every 5 minutes.
3. Allow the nuts to cool for 10 minutes.
4. In a high-powered blender, add nuts and additional ingredients. Process mixture until creamy. Coconut oil can be added in small amounts to help the blending process and texture.
5. Transfer nut butter into container and store in refrigerator.

Day Eight, Breakfast

Breakfast tacos are extremely satisfying and delicious. To make the Keto-Vegan tortillas, refer to the Fajita recipe on Day Three, lunch. If short on time, skip the tortillas and make this into a breakfast bowl. Additional toppings can include mushrooms, onions, peppers, avocado, walnut taco meat, and salsa.

Breakfast Tacos

Time: 20 minutes

Serving Size: 1 serving

Ingredients:

- 2-3 Keto tortillas (See Day 3, Lunch)
- ½ block firm tofu (7oz/200g)
- 1 tablespoon/14 grams nutritional yeast
- 1 tablespoon/25mL olive oil
- Pinch of turmeric powder
- Pinch of onion powder
- Himalayan salt and pepper to taste

Directions:

1. Prepare Keto tortillas.

2. In a large pan, smash the tofu into pieces using a spatula. Add in olive oil and remaining spices.
3. Cook the tofu eggs until little to no water is remaining.
4. Pour eggs into Keto tortillas.
5. Top tortillas with vegetables and dressing of choice.

Day Eight, Lunch

For today's lunch, prepare this delicious dressing and pour over greens. Kale, spinach, or arugula are all good options. Consider toppings like crushed nuts, tomato, cucumber, onion, olives, avocado, or peppers.

Cesar Salad

Time: 10 minutes

Serving Size: 3 servings

Ingredients:

- ½ cup/80 grams hemp hearts
- ½ cup/120mL water
- 2 tablespoons/30mL lemon juice
- 1 tablespoon/15mL mustard of choice
- 1 tablespoon/15mL coconut aminos
- 2 tablespoons/28 grams nutritional yeast
- 1 teaspoon/4 grams minced garlic
- 1 teaspoon/4 grams smoked paprika (optional)
- Sea salt and black pepper to preference

Directions:

1. In a blender, add all ingredients and pulse until everything is mixed well.
2. Pour dressing over salad with toppings of choice.

Day Eight, Dinner

Broccoli Cheddar Soup

Time: 25 minutes

Serving Size: 4 servings

Ingredients:

- 1 medium onion, chopped
- 3 teaspoons/14 grams garlic, minced
- 1 full broccoli head (2 cups/350 grams)
- 1 large carrot, chopped
- ½ teaspoon/2 grams turmeric
- 1 vegan bouillon cube
- 2 tablespoons/30mL olive oil
- ½ cup/65 grams raw cashews
- 2 tablespoons/28 grams nutritional yeast
- 2 tablespoons/30mL lemon juice
- 3¼ cups/750mL water
- Salt and pepper to preference

Directions:

1. In a small pot, bring water to a boil. Add cashews into pot and boil for 10 minutes.
2. If necessary, prepare broccoli by cutting into florets or small pieces.
3. In a pan, sauté onions using oil as necessary. Add garlic and sauté until onions are softened.
4. In a large pot, place broccoli, carrot, turmeric, and bouillon cube and bring the water to a boil. Cook for 10 minutes or until carrots are soft.
5. Drain cashews and place them into a blender along with the nutritional yeast. Pulse and blend until a smooth consistency appears. This can take up to five minutes depending on the strength of the blender.
6. Set the sauce into a bowl using a spatula if necessary.
7. When the vegetables are ready, transfer as much as possible to the same blender used before. Puree the soup. For optimal results, leave some broccoli and carrots whole to give some dimension to the soup.

8. Transfer everything back into the large pot and add remaining ingredients, any additional spices, and the cheese sauce. Allow everything to simmer for at least 10 minutes before serving.

Day Eight, Snack

These bombs are perfect for chocolate and mint lovers. Although the whole recipe takes about 40 minutes, the preparation time is super short and the recipe yields enough fat bombs for the full week!

Fat Bomb- Mint Chocolate Chip

Time: 40 minutes

Serving Size: 19 servings

Ingredients:

For the Filling
- ½ cup/118mL coconut butter, melted
- ½ cup/118 mL coconut oil, melted
- 1 teaspoon/2.5 mL peppermint extract
- ½ teaspoon/2 grams powdered stevia

Chocolate Coating
- ½ cup/64 grams cocoa powder
- ½ cup/118mL coconut oil melted
- ¾ teaspoon/3.5 grams powdered Stevia
- 1 teaspoon /5mL vanilla extract

Directions:

For the Filling
1. Combine all ingredients and mix thoroughly.
2. Using a tablespoon, fill an ice cube tray or mini muffin liners pouring 2 tablespoons (30mL) into each.
3. Freeze until solid.

For the Coating

4. Combine all ingredients and mix thoroughly.
5. Remove bombs from freezer and remove from tray or liner.
6. With a fork, place each bomb into the melted chocolate mixture. Place on parchment paper.
7. Continue until no bombs remain. Pour any additional chocolate coating over bombs.
8. Freeze solid and then store in the refrigerator in an airtight container.

Day Nine, Breakfast

Indulge in this sugar-free homemade jelly. The recipe below calls for blueberries but other berries or a combination can be used. Depending on how sweet the jelly is preferred, Stevia can be adjusted. For today's breakfast, smooth coconut oil and jelly over the Keto-Vegan bread. Recipe for bread is found on Day Two, Breakfast recipe.

Toast with Jelly

Time: 20 minutes

Serving Size: 10 servings

Ingredients:

- 2 slices Keto-Vegan Bread (See Day 2, Breakfast)
- 2 cups/200 grams blueberries
- ½ cup/125mL water
- 1 teaspoon/4 grams powdered Stevia
- 2 teaspoons/9mL lemon juice
- ½ teaspoon/2 grams lemon zest

Directions:

1. In a saucepan, add blueberries, water, and Stevia. Over medium heat, bring the mixture to simmer for four minutes.
2. As the blueberries become soft, mash using a fork.

3. Turn the heat to low and allow mixture to simmer for 10 minutes.
4. Add lemon juice and lemon zest. Stir well until powder is dissolved.
5. Turn off the heat and allow cooling before storing. Store in an airtight container or glass jar and refrigerate.

Day Nine, Lunch

For today's lunch, chop cucumbers, carrots, and avocado. With arugula, spring mix, romaine, spinach or any other lettuce, sprinkle toppings, dressing, green onion, and toasted sesame seeds for a Keto take on the sushi roll.

Sushi Salad- Dressing

Time: 15 minutes

Serving Size: 4 servings

Ingredients:

- 1 medium avocado
- 1 small lime, squeezed into juice
- 1 tablespoons/14 grams wasabi powder (optional)
- 2 tablespoons/30mL olive oil
- 2 teaspoons/9 mL rice vinegar (substitute: apple cider vinegar, regular)
- ½ teaspoon/3 grams garlic powder
- 1 thumb ginger or ½ teaspoon (3 grams)
- Sea salt and pepper to preference

Directions:

1. In a blender, add all ingredients and pulse until well mixed and creamy.
2. Taste and adjust wasabi or ginger levels.
3. Pour dressing over salad and add additional toppings.

Day Nine, Dinner

This recipe is a take on one of Britain's favorite dishes. Shepherd's pie is sure to comfort and add extra specialness to a cozy night. Spices and quantities of each vegetable or spice can be adjusted to your liking.

Shepherd's Pie

Time: 1 Hour

Serving Size: 2 servings

Ingredients:

- 1½ pound/325 grams cauliflower, in florets/pieces
- 2 tablespoon/30mL olive oil
- 1 small onion, diced
- 1 medium sized carrot, peeled and chopped
- 1 celery stalk, diced
- 2 teaspoons/8 grams of garlic, minced
- 2 cups/250 grams mushrooms, roughly chopped
- ½ tablespoon/7 grams thyme leaves, roughly chopped
- ½ tablespoon/7 grams tomato paste
- 3 tablespoons/45mL dry red wine
- ½ cup/120mL vegetable stock
- 1½ tablespoon/23 grams nutritional yeast
- ½ tablespoon/7 grams Dijon mustard
- ½ tablespoon/7 grams rosemary
- Pinch of nutmeg
- Himalayan salt and black pepper to taste

Directions:

1. Preheat oven to 400 degrees Fahrenheit or 200 degrees Celsius.
2. In a pot, bring water to a boil and cook cauliflower until tender. Drain the water when finished.
3. In a separate pan, add olive oil, onions, carrots, celery, and half of the mushrooms. Add the other half throughout the cooking to mix up the textures. Cook over medium heat until golden brown or caramelized.
4. Add tomato paste, vegetable stock, and red wine and stir.
5. Simmer for five to ten minutes or until liquid has mostly evaporated. Remove from heat.

6. Place cauliflower in a food processor along with nutritional yeast, mustard, thyme leaves, rosemary, nutmeg, pepper, and salt. Blend until smooth.
7. In two ramekins, divide the vegetable mixture and top with cauliflower.
8. Bake for 20 minutes or until lightly golden.

Day Nine, Snack

Carrot cake can still be enjoyed while on a Keto-Vegan diet. This recipe takes the traditional carrot cake and turns it into low calorie, low carb bites that can be enjoyed guilt-free!

Carrot Cake Bites

Time: 20 minutes

Serving Size: 15 servings

Ingredients:

- ½ cup/64 grams coconut flour
- ½ cup/237mL water
- 2 tablespoons/30mL applesauce, unsweetened
- ½ teaspoon/2 grams vanilla extract
- 1 teaspoon/4 grams nutmeg
- 1 teaspoon/4 grams cinnamon
- 1 tablespoon/15 grams powdered Stevia
- 1 medium carrot, shredded
- 4 tablespoons/60 grams shredded coconut, unsweetened

Directions:

1. In a large bowl combine coconut flour, water, applesauce, and vanilla extract.
1. Add in Stevia, nutmeg, cinnamon, and shredded carrots. Mix well.
2. Place mixture in refrigerator for 15 minutes.
3. Place shredded coconut into a separate bowl.
4. Remove dough from refrigerator and form into small balls. This recipe should yield about 15 bites.
5. Roll ball into shredded coconut and place into an airtight container. Store in refrigerator.

Day Ten, Breakfast

This breakfast is wonderful to make the night before a busy morning. Additional toppings can be added and nuts can be substituted with pecans, walnuts, Brazil nuts, almonds, cashews, or a mix. Blueberries can also be substituted for another Keto-friendly berry.

Overnight Oats

Time: 5 minutes

Serving Size: 2 servings

Ingredients:

- ⅔ cup/160mL full-fat coconut milk
- ½ cup/75 grams hemp hearts
- 1 tablespoon/15 grams chia seeds
- ½ teaspoon/2mL vanilla extract
- Pinch of sea salt
- Pinch of Stevia to preference
- ⅓ cup shredded coconut flakes, unsweetened
- 12 macadamia nuts
- 6 blueberries

Directions:

1. Add coconut milk, hemp hearts, chia seeds, vanilla, salt, and Stevia into a bowl and mix well.
2. Place bowl in refrigerator overnight.
3. In the morning, top with coconut flakes, macadamia nuts, blueberries and any other desired toppings.

Day Ten, Lunch

Today's lunch pairs perfectly with a Keto-Vegan tortilla, English muffin or bread. Sliced cucumbers and tomatoes can also be enjoyed with this egg salad. This recipe can also be enjoyed over a bed of lettuce with olive oil for an additional dressing.

Egg Salad

Time: 5 minutes

Serving Size: 4 servings

Ingredients:

- 1 block tofu, extra firm
- 1 stalk celery, diced
- 1 tablespoon/15mL coconut aminos
- 1½ tablespoons/23 grams nutritional yeast
- 1½ tablespoon/25 grams mustard
- 2 tablespoons/30 grams relish or chopped pickles (optional)
- ½ teaspoon/2 grams turmeric
- ¼ teaspoon/1 gram onion powder
- 1 tablespoon plant milk (almond, coconut, cashew, etc.)

Directions:

6. Drain tofu and press excess moisture using clean dish towel or paper towel. Place tofu in bowl.
7. Using a fork or hands, crumble tofu and finely as possible.
8. Mix in remaining ingredients and mix well. Store in refrigerator until ready to be consumed.

Day Ten, Dinner

For today's dinner, serve falafel over a salad or cooked cauliflower rice. Adjust spices as needed and to preference.

Falafel

Time: 25 minutes

Serving Size: 5 servings

Ingredients:

- 1 cup/225 grams lupini beans, rinsed well
- 3 tablespoons hemp hearts
- 3 tablespoons/45mL olive oil
- 3 tablespoons/45mL water
- 3 tablespoons/45 grams parsley, chopped
- 2 teaspoons/8 grams onion powder
- 2 teaspoons/8 grams garlic powder
- 2 teaspoons/9 mL hot sauce (optional)
- ½ teaspoon/2 grams baking powder
- ½ teaspoon/2 grams cumin
- ¼ teaspoon/1 gram paprika
- Himalayan salt and pepper to preference

Directions:

1. Preheat oven to 400 degrees Fahrenheit or 205 degrees Celsius. Line a baking sheet with parchment paper.
2. Place lupini beans in a blender or food processor and pulse until roughly chopped.
3. Add hemp hearts, olive oil, parsley, onion powder, garlic powder, and hot sauce. Pulse until smoothie. Add water as needed until mix becomes very smooth.
4. Transfer mixture to bowl and mix in remaining ingredients.
5. Form small falafel balls and place onto lined baking sheet.
6. Place in oven and bake for 16 to 19 minutes. Remove from oven and allow cooling. Store in airtight container and place in freezer or refrigerator until served.

Day Ten, Snack

Today's snack is wonderful on it's own or can also give extra flavor and crunchiness to other dishes. Sprinkle nuts over a salad or over a dessert. The nuts can be adjusted to preference. Walnuts, pecans, Brazil nuts, and peanuts are all great options. A mixture can be done as well.

Candied Nuts

Time: 12 minutes

Serving Size: 2 servings

Ingredients:

- 2 cups/440 grams unsalted cashews
- 1 cup/220 grams macadamia nuts
- 1 tablespoon/15 grams powdered Stevia (adjust as needed)
- 1 tablespoon/15 grams cinnamon (optional)
- ¼ cup/60 grams water
- 1 teaspoon/5mL vanilla extract
- ½ cup toasted coconut flakes
- Pinch of sea salt to preference

Directions:

1. Place a large frying pan over medium heat. Place nuts in pan and add sweetner, vanilla extract, and spices. Mix well.
2. Allow nuts to reach a golden brown color and remove from heat.
3. Allow cooling and sprinkle in coconut flakes.
4. Cool and store in airtight container.

Day Eleven, Breakfast

Today's breakfast is quick and easy. Substitute strawberries for any other Keto approved fruit or berry. If vegan protein is not available to you, consider adding in more almond butter or an avocado for extra fat and protein.

Breakfast Smoothie- Strawberry

Time: 5 minutes

Serving Size: 1 serving

Ingredients:

- 1 cup/237mL plant milk
- 1 scoop vegan protein powder (optional)
- ½ cup/110 grams strawberries, frozen
- 1 tablespoon/15 grams chia seeds
- 1 tablespoon/15mL coconut oil
- 1 teaspoon/4 grams powdered Stevia (to preference)
- 1 tablespoon/15 grams almond butter

Directions:

1. In a blender, place all ingredients and blend until smooth. Enjoy right away or cover and refrigerate.

Day Eleven, Lunch

Tomato soup is healthy, low calorie and very satisfying. This recipe can also be made in an instant pot. Place all ingredients in the pot and cook on high pressure for 5 minutes. Toasted nuts can be added as an additional topping!

Tomato Soup

Time: 20 minutes

Serving Size: 8 servings

Ingredients:

- 3.5 cups/328mL vegetable broth stock
- 1 medium onion
- 1 teaspoon/4 grams garlic, minced
- 1 teaspoon/4 grams oregano
- ½ teaspoon/2 grams smoked paprika
- 7 basil leaves
- 3 cans/400 grams diced or crushed tomatoes
- 1 teaspoon/4 grams cocoa powder, unsweetened
- Sea salt and pepper to taste

Directions:

1. Add all ingredients into a large pot.
2. Bring the pot to a boil and then reduce to low heat. Allow the soup to summer for 15 or 20 minutes until thick.
3. Soup can be placed in blender or eaten as is.

Day Eleven, Dinner

Today's dinner is filled with high nutrition and remains low in calories. If a grill is not available, use a medium saucepan and cook mushrooms until golden brown. This can be served over a bed of riced cauliflower if desired.

Grilled Portobello with Spinach

Time: 25 minutes

Serving Size: 4 servings

Ingredients:

- 4 large Portobello mushroom caps
- ¼ cup/60 mL olive oil
- 1 tablespoon/15mL red wine vinegar
- ½ cup/110 grams pecans
- 1⅓ cup/293 grams of frozen spinach
- 1 can/266mL coconut milk
- ½ small lemon
- Himalayan salt and pepper to taste

Directions:

1. Thaw out spinach and remove excess water.
2. Place spinach in saucepan and add coconut milk, salt, pepper, and a squeeze of lemon juice. Cook over medium heat until sauce is thick and creamy.
3. Allow the sauce to simmer on low heat and rest until the mushrooms are finished.
4. Scrape the black gills out of the mushrooms caps so they resemble a bowl.
5. Mix olive oil and vinegar together and coat both sides of the mushroom cap.
6. Set a grill to high heat. Set mushrooms on the grill and cook each side for about 5 minutes each.
7. Turn oven to broiler.
8. Fill the mushrooms with spinach and place under broiler for five minutes.
9. Serve mushrooms with chopped pecans and additional spices of choice.

Day Eleven, Snack

These are the perfect chips to curb any salty cravings. Below is the recipe for the chips and a recipe for taco seasoning. Store bought taco seasoning can contain sugar and extra, unhealthy ingredients that aren't natural.

Zucchini Chips- Taco Seasoning Recipe

Time: 10 minutes

Serving Size: 4 servings

Ingredients:

- 1 large zucchini
- Avocado oil, as needed
- Himalayan salt to preference
- 1 tablespoon taco seasoning
    - ☐ 2 tablespoons/30 grams ground chilli pepper
    - ☐ 1 tablespoon/15 grams cumin
    - ☐ 1 teaspoon/4 grams garlic powder
    - ☐ 1 teaspoon/4 grams onion powder
    - ☐ ½ tablespoon/8 grams paprika
    - ☐ 1 teaspoon/4 grams oregano
    - ☐ Pinch of cayenne pepper (optional)

Directions:

1. To create seasoning, mix all ingredients well in a bowl using a spoon. Store in airtight container in spice cabinet.
2. Cut the zucchini into thin chips. These strips should be as thin as possible.
3. Set chips aside into colander and remove as much excess water as possible from chips. Sprinkle with Himalayan salt and stir.
4. Place a generous amount of oil into the frying pan and turn to high heat.
5. Drop the chips into the hot oil. Once the chips turn golden brown remove and set chips onto paper towel to dry.
6. Sprinkle taco seasoning over chips and allow cooling. Store in airtight container.

Day Twelve, Breakfast

These Keto-Vegan bagels can be enjoyed with jelly, nut butter, coconut oil, or vegan cream cheese! They also can make great sandwich bread for breakfast or lunch.

Bagel

Time: 50 minutes

Serving Size: 6 servings

Ingredients:

- ½ cup/56 grams ground flax seeds
- ½ cup/112 grams tahini, unsalted
- ¼ cup/20 grams psyllium husks
- 1 cup/240mL water
- 1 teaspoon/4 grams baking powder
- Pinch of salt

Directions:

1. Preheat oven to 375 degrees Fahrenheit or 190 degrees Celsius.
2. In a bowl, mix psyllium husk, ground flax seeds, and baking powder. Mix well.
3. Add the water to the tahini and thoroughly whisk the two together.
4. Combine ingredients and knead the dough. Be sure that everything is mixed thoroughly.
5. Separate the dough into 6 even balls.
6. Take one ball and form a patty. Place patties on baking tray. A doughnut pan can also be used.
7. Cut a hole in each patty to resemble a bagel.
8. Bake for 40 minutes or until golden brown.
9. When ready to consume, cut bagel in half and place in toaster if desired.

Day Twelve, Lunch

Today's salad is super easy and will satisfy Mexican Cuisine lovers. If short on time, skip the sautéing and eat the vegetables as a raw salad.

Fajita Salad- Sour Cream Recipe

Time: 15 minutes

Serving Size: 4 serving

Ingredients:

For the Sour Cream
- 1 cup/220 grams raw cashews
- ½ cup/120mL water
- 1½ tablespoons/22mL apple cider vinegar
- ½ tablespoon/7mL lemon juice
- Sea salt to preference

For the Salad
- ½ avocado, peeled and pitted
- 1 red bell pepper, sliced
- 1 medium onion, chopped
- 1 cup/220 grams mushrooms
- 3 cups/500 grams lettuce of choice
- 1 small tomato, chopped
- 1 tablespoon/15mL olive oil

Directions:

1. In a small pot, bring water to a boil. Add cashews into boiling water and allow them to soak in the water for 10 minutes.
2. Drain the cashews and place into a high-speed blender with all other sour cream ingredients.
3. Blend until smooth and refrigerate until ready to be consumed. The sauce will thicken as it is chilled.
4. To make the rest of the salad, sauté the onion, red bell pepper, and mushrooms in a saucepan over medium heat. Add olive oil to prevent burning.
5. Pour sauteed vegetables over a bed of lettuce and top with avocado, tomato, and sour cream.

Day Twelve, Dinner

These buffalo bites are perfect for any time of the year and excellent for parties, special occasions, and sport games. Serve these bites with celery sticks and Vegan Ranch!

Buffalo Bites

Time: 50 minutes

Serving Size: 8 servings

Ingredients:

For the Bites
- 1 head of cauliflower (6 cups/2kg)
- ½ cup/120mL water
- ¼ cup/32 grams almond flour
- ¼ cup/32 grams tapioca flour
- 2 tablespoons/17 grams coconut flour
- ½ teaspoon/3 grams garlic powder

For the Buffalo Sauce
- ⅔ cup hot sauce of choice
- 2 tablespoons olive oil
- ½ teaspoon onion powder
- Sea salt and pepper to preference

Ranch Dip
- ⅔ cup/200grams vegan mayonnaise
- ⅓ cup/76 mL full-fat coconut milk
- 1 teaspoon/5mL apple cider vinegar
- ½ teaspoon/2 grams parsley
- ½ teaspoon/2 grams dill
- ½ teaspoon/2 grams of garlic powder
- ½ teaspoon/2 grams onion powder

Directions:

1. Preheat oven to 450 degrees Fahrenheit or 230 degrees Celsius. Line a baking sheet with parchment paper.
2. In a large bowl, whisk together water, almond flour, tapioca flour, coconut flour, and garlic powder.

3. Add in cauliflower florets and toss until each floret is covered in the batter. Place evenly on parchment paper.
4. Bake the cauliflower tor 20 minutes.
5. Combine hot sauce, olive oil, onion powder, salt, and pepper in a large bowl. Mix well.
6. Remove cauliflower from oven and add into buffalo sauce bowl. Toss cauliflower bites so they are evenly coated with sauce and return to parchment paper.
7. Bake for an additional 10 minutes before removing from oven. Serve bites immediately.
8. Place all ranch dressing ingredients into a bowl and mix well. Serve chilled.

Day Twelve, Snack

These coconut clusters make a great addition to ice cream, overnight oats, vegan yogurt, or for snacking. These clusters are perfect on the go and are even great with a splash of plant milk in the morning.

Coconut Clusters

Time: 15 minutes

Serving Size: 4 servings

Ingredients:

- 1½ cups/75 grams coconut flakes
- ½ cup/55 grams pepitas
- ½ cup/65 grams sunflower seeds
- 2 tablespoons/25 grams chia seeds
- 2 tablespoons/30mL coconut oil
- 1-2 tablespoons powdered Stevia
- 1 teaspoon vanilla extract
- 1 teaspoon/4 grams cinnamon (optional)
- Pinch of Himalayan salt

Directions:

1. Preheat oven to 350 degrees Fahrenheit or 175 degrees Celsius. Line a baking sheet with parchment paper.
2. Combine coconut flakes, pepitas, sunflower seeds, and chia seeds in a large bowl.
3. In a large saucepan, melt coconut oil, cinnamon, vanilla, Stevia and salt over medium heat.
4. Add the nuts to the saucepan and stir well before pouring mixture onto lined baking sheet.
5. Bake for 5-10 minutes until coconut flakes are golden brown.
6. Remove pan and allow some time for cooling. Break mixture into clusters and store in an airtight container.

Day Thirteen, Breakfast

This recipe takes less than five minutes to prepare and is best stored overnight. Prepare this recipe the night before and enjoy on the go during a quick morning. Garnish the top with an extra scoop of nut butter, coconut clusters, and Stevia sweetened vegan chocolate chips if desired.

Chocolate Pudding

Time: 1 hour

Serving Size: 6 servings

Ingredients:

- 1 cup/220 grams ground chia seeds
- 3 tablespoons/45 grams cocoa powder, unsweetened
- 2 cups/440 grams coconut milk
- 2 tablespoons/30 grams peanut butter
- 1 tablespoon/15 grams powdered Stevia
- ½ teaspoon/3mL vanilla extract
- Pinch of sea salt

Directions:

1. In a blender, blend all ingredients until smooth. Blend for an additional minute after everything is smooth.

2. Taste the mixture and adjust sweetness levels.
3. Transfer mixture into a jar or airtight container using a spatula if needed.
4. Store in refrigerator for one hour before serving to thicken pudding.
5. When ready to consume, top with desired toppings.

Day Thirteen, Lunch

This pasta salad is perfect for a light lunch or a perfect side to share with others. This recipe can be served hot or cold.

Pasta Salad

Time: 10 minutes

Serving Size: 2 servings

Ingredients:

- 1 large, seeded and peeled cucumber, spiralized
- 1 medium zucchini, spiralized
- 1 cup olives of choice
- 1 small tomato, sliced
- 1 small red onion, chopped
- ½ cup/170 grams vegan feta (See Day 4, Lunch)
- ⅓ cup/120 grams red pepper, chopped
- ½ avocado, peeled and pitted
- 4 tablespoons/60mL olive oil
- 2 tablespoons/30mL apple cider vinegar
- Sea salt and black pepper to preference

Directions:

1. Add spiralized zucchini and cucumber into a large bowl.
2. Add olives, tomato, onion, feta, red pepper, and avocado.
3. Add in salt, pepper, olive oil, and apple cider vinegar. Mix well. Refrigerate until served.

Day Thirteen, Dinner

This recipe takes less than 10 minutes of preparation and little effort. Throw this in the slow cooker during a lunch break or on a weekend. An instant pot can also be used.

Rice and Beans

Time: 4 hours

Serving Size: 6 servings

Ingredients:

- 2 packages cauliflower rice, frozen (24 oz./340g)
- 2 cans black soy beans, rinsed and drained
- ½ cup/80 grams hulled hemp seeds
- 1 cup/237mL vegetable broth
- 3 tablespoons/45mL avocado oil
- 2⅓ tablespoons/35 grams taco seasoning (See Day 11, Snack)

Toppings
- ½ avocado, peeled and pitted
- 1 medium tomato, sliced
- Vegan sour cream (See Day 12, Lunch)
- 1 small red onion, chopped

Directions:

1. Add all ingredients excluding the toppings to a slow cooker. Mix well.
2. Allow the mixture to cook for three to four hours until the rice is tender.
3. Serve and garnish with toppings.

Day Thirteen, Snack

This recipe is a great dessert for after a long day. Consider melting Stevia sweetened, vegan chocolate over the top and sprinkling with a few nuts.

Almond Flour Blondies

Time: 20 minutes

Serving Size: 16 servings

Ingredients:

- 2 cups/256 grams blanched almond flour
- 1 tablespoon/15 grams powdered Stevia
- 2 tablespoons/20 grams coconut flour
- 1 teaspoon/4 grams baking powder
- ¼ cup/60mL water
- Pinch of sea salt

Directions:

1. Preheat oven to 350 degrees Fahrenheit or 175 degrees Celsius. Line a baking sheet with parchment paper.
2. In a bowl, mix almond flour, coconut flour, Stevia, baking powder, and salt. Add water slowly and mix until well blended.
3. Press the dough onto the parchment paper forming a rectangle. Smooth the top.
4. Bake for 16 to 20 minutes or until edges are golden brown.
5. Remove from oven and allow cooling. Cut into about 16 bars and store in an airtight container.

Day Fourteen, Breakfast

Serve this delicious bread with melted coconut oil, nut butter, or homemade jelly.

Keto Pumpkin Bread

Time: 1 hour

Serving Size: 1 loaf, 10 slices

Ingredients:

- ⅓ cup/80mL almond milk, unsweetened
- 2 tablespoons/25 grams powdered Stevia
- 2 tablespoons/14 grams flax seeds
- 1 teaspoon/5mL vanilla extract
- ¾ cup/170 grams pumpkin puree
- ½ cup/112 grams coconut oil, softened
- 1¼ cup/160 grams coconut flour
- 1 teaspoon/4 grams cinnamon
- 1 teaspoon/4 grams nutmeg
- ½ teaspoon/4 grams baking powder
- ¼ teaspoon/2 grams baking soda
- Pinch of Himalayan salt

Directions:

1. Preheat oven to 350 degrees Fahrenheit or 177 degrees Celsius. Line a loaf pan with parchment paper. Leave the parchment paper long at the sides for easy removal later.
2. In a bowl, mix almond milk, Stevia, flax seeds, and vanilla. Mix well and set aside for 5 minutes.
3. Stir in pumpkin puree and coconut oil.
4. In a separate bowl, mix coconut flour, cinnamon, nutmeg, baking powder, baking soda, and salt. Mix well.
5. Combine both mixtures and mix well.
6. Pour batter into the loaf pan and bake for 50 minutes. When a toothpick comes out clean from the center, the loaf is complete.
7. Remove loaf pan from oven and let the bread cool before cutting into about 10 slices.

Day Fourteen, Lunch

Today's lunch is a great recipe to serve over a bed of lettuce, between two slices of Keto bread, with celery stalks, or with Keto-Vegan crackers. If kelp powder is not available to you, substitute with nutritional yeast or seaweed crackers (sold in most stores).

Tuna Salad

Time: 10 minutes

Serving Size: 4 servings

Ingredients:

- 1 block extra firm tofu
- ½ cup vegan mayo
- 2 celery stalks, chopped
- 1 carrot, chopped
- ½ teaspoon kelp powder
- 1 teaspoon/4 grams onion powder
- 1 teaspoon/5mL lemon juice
- Sea salt and pepper to preference

Directions:

1. Drain and remove excess water from tofu.
2. In a bowl, crumble the tofu using hands or a fork.
3. Add in the remaining ingredients and mix well.
4. Store any leftovers in an airtight container in the refrigerator.

Day Fourteen, Dinner

This recipe is an impressive dish that can be eaten as a side or meal. Not only does the dish looks beautiful, but it tastes good too! Turn Keto bread into garlic toast and serve alongside this dish for a complete meal.

Zucchini Tomato Bake

Time: 45 minutes

Serving Size: 4 servings

Ingredients:

For the Sauce
- 1 cup/220 grams fresh basil leaves
- 1 tablespoon/15 grams pepitas
- 2 teaspoons/30 grams garlic, minced
- 2 tablespoons/30mL olive oil
- 1 tablespoon/15mL water
- Himalayan salt and pepper to preference

Vegetables
- 1 tablespoon avocado oil
- 3 medium zucchini
- 2 small onions
- 2 medium tomatoes
- ½ teaspoon/2 grams oregano
- 1 teaspoon/4 grams red pepper flakes (optional)

Directions:

1. Preheat oven to 350 degrees Fahrenheit or 175 degrees Celsius.
2. After washing vegetables, use a mandoline to slice zucchini, onions, and tomatoes as thin as possible. Use a sharp knife if a mandolin is not available.
3. In a cast iron pan, distribute avocado oil.
4. Arrange veggies in the pan alternating between zucchini, onion, and tomatoes. Arrange the veggies in a spiral pattern. Do not lay veggies flat, but standing up.
5. In a blender, place all sauce ingredients and blend until smooth.
6. Pour the sauce over the veggies. Save a little for after.
7. Cover the pan with parchment paper to prevent burning and bake for 30 minutes or until the veggies are soft.

8. Pour the remaining sauce over the vegetables and serve.

Day Fourteen, Snack

Cookie dough is a household favorite for many. Not only is this recipe eggless, it's vegan and low carb! These bites can also be made smaller and be used as a topping on other desserts like ice cream!

Edible Cookie Dough

Time: 5 minutes

Serving Size: 16 bites

Ingredients:

- 1 cup/128 grams almond flour
- ¼ cup/32 grams coconut flour
- 2 tablespoons/25 grams powdered Stevia
- 3 tablespoons/45mL coconut oil, melted
- ¼ cup/60 grams coconut cream
- 1 tablespoon/15mL vanilla extract
- ¼ cup/45 grams vegan, stevia sweetened chocolate chips
- 2 tablespoons/30mL coconut milk, unsweetened
- Pinch of sea salt

Directions:

1. In a bowl, mix almond flour, coconut flour, and a pinch of sea salt.
2. Add coconut oil, coconut cream, and vanilla. Mix well.
3. Add coconut milk to make the batter creamy.
4. Add in chocolate chips.
5. Roll the batter into about 16 bites and store in refrigerator.

Day Fifteen, Breakfast

Today's recipe combines a few recipes in this guide and puts them into a burrito. The tortilla recipe can be found on Day 3, lunch. Not listed is the additional toppings. Consider adding avocado, mushrooms, and tomatoes to the burrito. This recipe can also be used for lunch. Omit the eggs and replace them with riced cauliflower.

Breakfast Burrito- Mild Salsa Recipe

Time: 20 minutes

Serving Size: 3 serving

Ingredients:

For the Burrito
- 4 Tortillas (See Day 3, Lunch)
- 8 ounces/220 grams extra firm tofu
- 1 tablespoon/15mL olive oil
- 2 tablespoon/30 grams nutritional yeast
- 1 tablespoon/15 grams onion powder
- ½ teaspoon/4 grams turmeric
- ⅓ cup/80mL almond milk
- Salt and black pepper to preference
- Hot sauce of choice (optional)

For the Salsa
- 2 large tomatoes, diced
- 1/4 medium red onion, finely chopped
- 1 teaspoon/4 grams garlic, minced
- 1 red chili, finely chopped
- ½ lime, juiced
- 1 tablespoon/15 grams cilantro, finely chopped
- 2 tablespoons/30mL olive oil
- Himalayan salt and pepper to preference

Directions:

1. Prepare the tortillas and set aside.
2. Prepare the eggs by removing as much excess water as possible and placing in a saucepan over medium heat. Crumble the tofu using a fork or spatula.
3. Add all other egg ingredients and cook the tofu for 4-5 minutes until an egg like texture forms.
4. Place eggs, and all other desired toppings into the tortillas.
5. In a bowl, mix all salsa ingredients together and refrigerate until ready to be served.

Day Fifteen, Lunch

This soup takes little to no effort and is great for fat burning. This recipe is also similar to chicken noodle soup and has great properties to boost the immune system.

Cabbage Soup

Time: 35 minutes

Serving Size: 8 servings

Ingredients:

- 1 large onion, chopped
- 1 large carrot, chopped
- 2 celery stalks, diced
- 3 teaspoons/15 grams garlic, minced
- ½ cup/110 grams parsley
- ¼ large cabbage
- 8 cups/1,880mL water
- 2 bouillon cubes, vegan
- 2 tablespoons/30mL avocado oil
- Salt and pepper to taste

Directions:

1. In a large pot, heat up avocado oil and place chopped onion, carrot, celery, and garlic inside. Cook until vegetables are soft.
2. Add water and bouillon cubes. Bring water to a boil.
3. Add in cabbage, parsley, and spiced. Stir.
4. Allow soup to simmer on low for 35 minutes.

Day Fifteen, Dinner

This recipe is perfect for the whole family. Simple and delicious, this recipe gives a healthy alternative French fry recipe. Consider serving the ranch sauce found Day Twelve, dinner.

Kebabs with Fries

Time: 45 minutes

Serving Size: 8 kebabs, 2 servings

Ingredients:

For the Kebabs
- 1 package firm tofu
- 1 medium red onion, sliced
- 2 bell peppers, sliced
- 2 small zucchini, sliced thick
- ¼ cup/60mL coconut aminos
- ¼ cup/40mL avocado oil
- ¼ cup/60mL apple cider vinegar
- 1 teaspoon/5mL liquid smoke (optional)
- 2 teaspoons/8 grams garlic, minced
- Sea salt and pepper to preference

For the Fries
- 2 medium zucchinis, cut into fries

- 2 tablespoons/17 grams almond flour
- ¼ cup/32 grams cup blanched almond flour
- 1 tablespoon/15 grams nutritional yeast
- 1 teaspoon/4 grams oregano
- Himalayan salt and pepper to preference

Directions:

1. Preheat oven to 450 degrees Fahrenheit or 232 degrees Celsius. Line a large baking sheet with parchment paper.
2. Preheat grill to 450 degrees Fahrenheit or 232 degrees Celsius. Brush the grate with oil.
3. Remove excess water from tofu by pressing with a clean dish towel or paper towels. Cut into square cubes, about one inch wide. Set aside.
4. In a bowl, whisk together coconut aminos, avocado oil, apple cider vinegar, garlic powder, liquid smoke, and salt and pepper. Set extra marinade aside for vegetables.
5. Place the tofu in the marinade bowl. Cover the tofu and allow the marinade to sink in. Allowing tofu to marinade overnight or for a few hours is best if possible.
6. In a large bowl, place zucchini fries along with almond milk.
7. Combine dry ingredients for fries (almond flour, nutritional yeast, and spices) in a large Ziploc bag.
8. Add zucchini into bag with seasonings and shake until evenly coated.
9. Place on lined baking sheet and cook for 20 minutes.
10. Remove fries from oven and flip the fries using a spatula. Bake fries for an additional 5-8 minutes or until golden brown.
11. Place all kebab vegetables into a bowl and toss with marinade.
12. Place vegetables and tofu pieces onto a skewer alternating vegetables and tofu.
13. Place skewers on the grill and cook for 15 minutes turning the skewers throughout. Both sides of the skewer should be firm with a few grill marks.

Day Fifteen, Snack

This recipe is another example of how modern foods can be made into healthy, delicious treats with just a few modifications! These brownies are perfect for the whole family and are sure to be popular at any party or get-together!

Brownies

Time: 45 minutes

Serving Size: 14 brownies

Ingredients:

- ¼ cup/56 grams chia seeds
- ¾ cup/177.5mL water
- 1 cup/225 grams pumpkin puree
- 1 cup/150 grams mashed avocado
- 2 cups/200 grams cocoa powder, unsweetened
- 6 tablespoons/50 grams coconut flour
- 1 tablespoon/8 grams baking soda
- ½ cup/125mL almond milk
- 1½ tablespoon/15 grams powdered Stevia
- ½ cup/75 grams vegan, Stevia sweetened chocolate chips

Directions:

1. Mix chia seeds with water and set aside for 20 minutes. A gel-like substance should form.
2. Preheat oven to 350 degrees Fahrenheit or 180 degrees Celsius. Line a baking 8 x 8 inch pan with parchment paper.
3. Place all other ingredients in a blender excluding the chocolate chips and almond milk. Blend well.
4. Add coconut milk and chocolate chips and pulse. Be careful to not blend the chocolate chips.
5. Pour the batter into the lined pan.
6. Bake for 30-35 minutes or until toothpick comes out clean from the center.
7. Allow cooling before slicing brownies.

Day Sixteen, Breakfast

This recipe pairs perfectly with keto-vegan eggs, breakfast tacos, breakfast burritos, or even for a side dish!

Hash Brown Patties

Time: 15 minutes

Serving Size: 2 servings

Ingredients:

- ½ head of cauliflower, in florets
- 1 tablespoon/15mL olive oil
- ½ medium onion, chopped
- ¼ cup/32 grams almond flour
- 1 tablespoon/8 grams cornstarch
- ½ teaspoon/3 grams garlic powder
- 2 tablespoons/30mL water
- Himalayan salt and pepper to preference

Directions:

1. Preheat oven to 400 degrees Fahrenheit or 205 degrees Celsius. Line a baking sheet with parchment paper. Grease parchment paper lightly with oil.
2. Using a food processor or grater, process cauliflower and onion until they appear like rice.
3. In a large bowl, add riced cauliflower, onion, almond flour, cornstarch, garlic powder, salt, and water and mix well.
4. Divide the dough into six equal portions and form patties.
5. Place patties onto greased, lined baking sheet and bake for 20 minutes.
6. Remove the baking sheet and flip the patties.
7. Allow an additional 20 minutes of baking or until crispy brown.

Day Sixteen, Lunch

Today's recipe combines two other recipes in this cookbook: candied nuts and vegan feta cheese. If short on time, omit the cheese and use regular nuts. Remember that fruits should be consumed in a small amount. After this meal, save the next berry snack for another day.

Spinach Salad with Berries

Time: 5 minutes

Serving Size: 1 salad

Ingredients:

- 3 cups/225 grams raw spinach
- ½ cup/100 grams strawberries
- ¼ cup candied nuts (Day 10, Snack)
- ⅓ cup/45 grams vegan feta cheese (Day 4, Lunch)

For the Dressing
- ½ cup apple cider vinegar
- ½ cup olive oil
- 2 teaspoons/8 grams garlic, minced
- Sea salt and pepper to preference

Directions:

1. Wash or prepare spinach, strawberries, nuts, and cheese in a bowl.
2. In a separate bowl or using a blender, combine all dressing ingredients.
3. Pour dressing over salad and mix well. Refrigerate until ready to be consumed.

Day Sixteen, Dinner

This savory dish will leave you feeling full and satisfied! Depending on how spicy you prefer your curry, red pepper flakes are optional. This dish can be made with any other Keto approved vegetables so get creative!

Red Curry

Time: 30 minutes

Serving Size: 3 servings

Ingredients:

- 2 large carrots, peeled and sliced
- ½ medium red bell pepper, sliced
- 1 small yellow squash, chopped
- 2 medium zucchini, spiralized
- 1 small lime, in wedges
- 3 green onions, chopped
- Fresh cilantro, chopped
- Sea salt and black pepper to preference

For the Sauce:
- 1 can coconut milk, full fat (14oz/415mL)
- 2 tablespoons/32 grams red curry paste
- 2 teaspoons/3.5 grams fresh ginger, grated
- 2 tablespoons/30mL coconut aminos
- 1 teaspoon/4 grams red pepper flakes (optional)
- 1 teaspoon/2 grams powdered Stevia

Directions:

1. In a large skillet, place all ingredients for the sauce over medium heat. Bring to a gentle boil and then reduce heat to low. Allow the sauce to simmer for 8 to 10 minutes. The sauce should thicken.
2. Prepare and chop vegetables.
3. Bring sauce to medium heat and add the carrots and bell peppers. Allow the vegetables to soften.
4. Add in zucchini and yellow squash. Stir well.
5. Cook the squash for three to five minutes. Do not overcook, or the squash will be soggy.

6. Remove the dish and serve with lime, green onions, cilantro, sea salt, and pepper.

Day Sixteen, Snack

Cookie dough is a household favorite for many. Not only is this recipe eggless, it's vegan and low carb! These bites can also be made smaller and be used as a topping on other desserts like ice cream!

Peanut Butter Bark

Time*:* 5 minutes

Serving Size: 2 servings

Ingredients:

- ¼ cup natural/65 grams organic peanut butter (no sugar added)
- ¼ cup/55 grams coconut oil
- 1 teaspoon/5mL vanilla extract
- 1 cup/115 grams chopped pecans
- Pinch of powdered Stevia
- 1 ounce/28.5 grams vegan, Stevia sweetened dark chocolate
- 1 teaspoon/5mL coconut oil
- Pinch of Himalayan salt

Directions:

1. Line two plates with parchment paper.
2. Melt the peanut butter and ¼ cup (55 grams) coconut oil in a bowl for 30 seconds or until melted.
3. Add in vanilla, stevia, pecans, and salt. Stir well.
4. Pour half of the mixture onto each plate and freeze.
5. Take the chocolate and 1 teaspoon (5mL) coconut oil and melt in microwave. This should take around 20 seconds. Be careful not to burn the chocolate.
6. Once the chocolate is frozen onto the plates, pour the chocolate over the top create a chocolate drizzle.
7. Store in freezer or refrigerator. Transfer the parchment paper into an airtight container.

Day Seventeen, Breakfast

This recipe is a take on cereal and is packed with fats and nutrients. This recipe makes for a great snack on the go, or for breakfast. Mix in your favorite plant milk and enjoy as cereal!

Cereal

Time: 35 minutes

Serving Size: 10 servings

Ingredients:

- 1 cup coconut flakes
- ½ cup cashews, chopped
- ½ pecans, chopped
- ½ cup macadamia nuts, chopped
- ½ cup sunflower seeds
- ½ cup pumpkin seeds
- 2 tablespoons chia seeds
- 2 tablespoons flaxseed meal
- ½ cup sliced almonds
- 1 teaspoon cinnamon (optional)
- Pinch of Himalayan salt
- 3 tablespoons coconut oil
- 1 teaspoon vanilla extract
- ½ cup freeze dried raspberries
- 2 tablespoons Stevia or to preference

Directions:

1. Preheat oven to 300 degrees Fahrenheit or 150 degrees Celsius. Line a baking sheet with parchment paper. Set aside.
2. In a large bowl mix coconut flakes, cashews, pecans, macadamia nuts, sunflower seeds, pumpkin seeds, chia seeds, almonds, flaxseed meal, cinnamon, and salt.
3. In a saucepan melt coconut oil with vanilla and sweetener over medium heat.
4. Combine the nut mixture and the sauce. Mix evenly.
5. Spread the mixture on the lined baking sheet and bake for 25 minutes. Stir halfway through. The mixture is done when everything is golden brown and crisp.
6. Remove the baking sheet from the oven and allow cooling. Stir in the dried raspberries.

7. Store in a glass jar or airtight container.

Day Seventeen, Lunch

Today's lunch is simple and quick. If short on time, omit the bagel and make this into a salad or emit the egg salad and double the avocado amount. Other Keto-approved vegetables are welcomed along with any other preferred Keto-Vegan dressing.

Bagel Sandwich

Time: 10 minutes

Serving Size: 1 serving

Ingredients:

- 1 bagel (Day 12, breakfast)
- 1 tablespoon yellow mustard
- 1 tablespoon vegan mayonnaise (optional)
- Handful of lettuce
- ¼ cucumber, sliced thin
- ½ avocado, mashed
- Handful of sprouts
- ½ cup egg salad (Day 10, lunch)

Directions:

1. Assemble the sandwich by washing and slicing vegetables.

Day Seventeen, Dinner

These nuggets are a great comfort food, and filling. Freezing and thawing the tofu gives it a meat-like texture that many people enjoy. If you're short on time, you can skip this step, but the nuggets won't be as chewy. Easy to make, they are also great the next day for a quick snack. Serve with the Keto-Vegan ranch dressing, or any other Keto-Vegan friendly sauce.

Chicken Nuggets with Ranch

Time: 35 minutes

Serving Size: 2 servings

Ingredients:

- 1 package extra firm tofu (12 oz./340 grams)
- 2 cup/475mL vegetable broth
- ⅓ cup/43 grams almond flour
- 2 tablespoons/30 grams nutritional yeast
- Himalayan salt and pepper to preference
- Ranch dressing (Day 12, dinner)

Directions:

1. Drain tofu and freeze for eight hours in an airtight container.
2. Remove tofu and allow the tofu to thaw out. Remove as much water as possible using a clean dishtowel or paper towels.
3. Cut tofu into chicken nuggets (bite sized pieces).
4. Place tofu into a bowl and cover with vegetable broth. Allow this to marinate as long as possible. Up to 4 hours if possible.
5. Preheat oven to 400 degrees Fahrenheit or 205 degrees Celsius. Line a baking sheet with parchment paper.
6. In a bowl, mix flour, nutritional yeast, salt, and pepper.
7. Place each tofu nugget in the mixture, coating it completely. Place onto parchment paper.
8. Bake for 10 minutes.
9. Remove pan and flip over each nugget. Bake for an additional 10-12 minutes or until the squares are brown and crispy.
10. Prepare ranch-dipping sauce.

Conclusion

The Keto-Vegan lifestyle is the healthiest diet out there. Both diets combine high fat and incredibly nutritious food, while omitting harmful foods that the body doesn't need.

The benefits that come along with the Keto-Vegan diet are extensive. While both physical and internal changes occur, the environment changes as well. Animal cruelty stops, and carbon emissions go down. Studies have shown the powerful impact the meat and dairy industry has on the world. To recap some of the statistics, a car would have to drive 250km (155 miles) to produce the same amount of pollution as 1 kg (2.2lbs) of beef. One kilogram of steak requires 18,000 liters (4,800 gallons) of water. The meat industry accounts for 75% of all farmland in the world while producing less than a third of daily calories. And lastly, switching to a vegan lifestyle reduces your personal carbon footprint by up to 73%. These statistics are alarming and the solution is a vegan lifestyle.

Not only will your overall appearance approve, but your body tone and shape as well. On the inside, cells and organs become stronger, and healthier than ever. Studies have proven time and time again that the Keto-Vegan diet not only protects against disease and cancers, but also has the capability of reversing them.

To recap some of the studies, one study with 200 patients had the participants switch to a plant based diet. Of these participants, 22% of the patients experienced a reversal in heart diseases and symptoms. This study was not surprising as a different study proved that cancer incidence is 20% lower in vegans. This is because a daily intake of red meat, mostly processed, increases the risk of heart disease by 42%. This is a problem as in the UK, every 5 minutes someone is admitted to the hospital for a heart attack. In the UK alone, 28% of people are dealing with heart disease. In addition to heart disease, the Keto-Vegan diet can also prevent and reverse diabetes.

Along with preventing and reversing disease, studies have shown that DNA compounds are better supported in a vegan lifestyle. Aging effects slow down and the body receives more vital nutrients. These anti-aging effects happen internally and are shown physically.

In regards to the Keto diet, implementing the diet alongside a vegan diet is powerful. Increasing fats and eliminating carbs and sugar are another reason why diseases and cancer risk are lower on this combined diet. Fat encourages a new energy source that replaces glucose. Ketone bodies are preferred by the body and brain and will aid in weight loss and cellular rejuvenation. Intermittent fasting alongside the Keto-Vegan diet is extremely helpful for weight loss. Working up to the preferred 16-8 method will greatly affect cells, weight loss, and overall health.

With all of these alarming statistics and studies proving the effectiveness of the Keto-Vegan diet, it's time for a change. Make the change for yourself, and know that your body, the environment, and animals will all benefit. Implementing a Keto-Vegan lifestyle is easy and the same foods can be enjoyed with healthy moderation!

Bibliography

A more potent greenhouse gas than carbon dioxide, methane emissions will leap as Earth warms. (2014, March 27). Retrieved from https://www.sciencedaily.com/releases/2014/03/140327111724.htm.

A Quarter of Brits Will be Vegan by 2025 and Half will be Flexitarian - economist - the vegan business magazine. (2019, May 24). Retrieved from https://vegconomist.com/studies-and-numbers/a-quarter-of-brits-will-be-vegan-by-2025-and-half-will-be-flexitarian/.

Berg, E. [Dr. Eric Berg DC]. (2017, May 9). What is Insulin Resistance? [Video file]. Retrieved from https://www.youtube.com/watch?v=pxl8hhyN6AQ

Berry, J. (2019, January 21). The 6 best benefits of macadamia nuts. Retrieved from https://www.medicalnewstoday.com/articles/324233.php.

Boyles, S. (2010, May 17). Processed Meat Linked to Heart, Diabetes Risks. Retrieved from https://www.webmd.com/heart-disease/news/20100517/processed-meat-linked-to-heart-disease-risks.

Brechon, S. (2013, September 6). Estrogen And Breast Cancer. Retrieved from https://www.maurerfoundation.org/estrogen-and-breast-cancer/.

British Heart Foundation. (2018, April 6). Can a plant-based diet 'reverse' heart disease? Retrieved from https://www.bhf.org.uk/informationsupport/heart-matters-magazine/nutrition/ask-the-expert/plant-based-diets.

Carrington, D. (2019, March 18). England could run short of water within 25 years. Retrieved from https://www.theguardian.com/environment/2019/mar/18/england-to-run-short-of-water-within-25-years-environment-agency.

Chi, M.-Y., M., Schlein, L., A., Moley, & H., K. (2000, December 1). High Insulin-Like Growth Factor 1 (IGF-1) and Insulin Concentrations Trigger Apoptosis in the Mouse Blastocyst via Down-Regulation of the IGF-1 Receptor * * This work was supported in part by NIH through Grants RO1-HD-38061–01A1 (to K.H.M.), P60-DK-30579 (to K.H.M.), and the Washington University Clinical Nutrition Research Unit Center Grant P30-DK-56341 (to K.H.M.); and by the Burroughs Wellcome Fund through a Career Award in the Biomedical Sciences (to K.H.M.). Retrieved from https://academic.oup.com/endo/article/141/12/4784/2988691.

Coote, S., & Sadeghi MD, A. (2017, June 20). Diabetes - Cause, Prevention, Treatment and Reversal with a Plant Based Diet. Retrieved from https://www.riseofthevegan.com/blog/diabetes-reversal-with-plant-based-diet.

Cruelty to Cows: How Cows Are Abused for Meat and Dairy Products: Animals Used for Food: Issues. (n.d.). Retrieved from https://www.petaasia.com/issues/food/cows/.

Current World Population. (n.d.). Retrieved from https://www.worldometers.info/world-population/.

Dolson, L. (2019, July 17). Why Your Body Needs Glycogen. Retrieved from https://www.verywellfit.com/what-is-glycogen-2242008.

Eating meat linked to higher risk of diabetes. (2017, September 5). Retrieved from https://www.sciencedaily.com/releases/2017/09/170905134506.htm.

Facts & Figures. (n.d.). Retrieved from https://www.diabetes.org.uk/professionals/position-statements-reports/statistics.

Facts and figures. (2019). Retrieved from https://www.bhf.org.uk/for-professionals/press-centre/facts-and-figures.

Ford, J. H. (2010, June). Saturated fatty acid metabolism is the key link between cell division, cancer, and senescence in cellular and whole organism aging. Retrieved from https://www.ncbi.nlm.nih.gov/pubmed/20431990.

Gunnars, K. (2018, January 11). Top 10 Evidence-Based Health Benefits of Coconut Oil. Retrieved from https://www.healthline.com/nutrition/top-10-evidence-based-health-benefits-of-coconut-oil.

History. (n.d.). Retrieved from https://www.vegansociety.com/about-us/history

Key, T. J., Appleby, P. N., Crowe, F. L., Bradbury, K. E., Schmidt, J. A., & Travis, R. C. (2014, July). Cancer in British vegetarians: updated analyses of 4998 incident cancers in a cohort of 32,491 meat eaters, 8612 fish eaters, 18,298 vegetarians, and 2246 vegans. Retrieved from https://www.ncbi.nlm.nih.gov/pubmed/24898235.

Leech, J. (2018, September 14). 11 Proven Benefits of Olive Oil. Retrieved from https://www.healthline.com/nutrition/11-proven-benefits-of-olive-oil#section1.

Livestock a major threat to environment. (2006, November). Retrieved from http://www.fao.org/newsroom/en/news/2006/1000448/index.html.

Lutas, A., & Yellen, G. (2013, January). The ketogenic diet: metabolic influences on brain excitability and epilepsy. Retrieved from https://www.ncbi.nlm.nih.gov/pubmed/23228828.

Mason, C., Risques, R.-A., Xiao, L., Duggan, C. R., Imayama, I., Campbell, K. L., … McTiernan, A. (2013, December). Independent and combined effects of dietary weight loss and exercise on leukocyte telomere length in postmenopausal women. Retrieved from https://www.ncbi.nlm.nih.gov/pmc/articles/PMC3786031/.

Moro, T., Marcolin, Battaglia, G., & Paoli, A. (2016, October 13). Effects of eight weeks of time-restricted feeding (16/8) on basal metabolism, maximal strength, body composition, inflammation, and cardiovascular risk factors in resistance-trained males. Retrieved from https://translational-medicine.biomedcentral.com/articles/10.1186/s12967-016-1044-0.

National Diabetes Statistics Report. (2018, February 24). Retrieved from https://www.cdc.gov/diabetes/data/statistics/statistics-report.html?CDC_AA_refVal=https://www.cdc.gov/diabetes/data/statistics/2014statisticsreport.html.

National Research Council (US) Committee on Diet, Nutrition, & Cancer, and. (1982, January 1). 13 Mutagens in Food. Retrieved from https://www.ncbi.nlm.nih.gov/books/NBK216630/.

Noh, H. S., Lee, H. P., Kim, D. W., Kang, S. S., Cho, G. J., Rho, J. M., & Choi, W. S. (2004, October 22). A cDNA microarray analysis of gene expression profiles in rat hippocampus following a ketogenic diet. Retrieved from https://www.ncbi.nlm.nih.gov/pubmed/15469884.

Ogino, A., Orito, H., Shimada, K., & Hirooka, H. (2007). Evaluating environmental impacts of the Japanese beef cow?calf system by the life cycle assessment method. Animal Science Journal, 78(4), 424–432. doi: 10.1111/j.1740-0929.2007.00457.x

Ornish, D., Lin, J., Daubenmier, J., Weidner, G., Epel, E., Kemp, C., … Blackburn, E. H. (2008). Increased telomerase activity and comprehensive lifestyle changes: a pilot study. The Lancet Oncology, 9(11), 1048–1057. doi: 10.1016/s1470-2045(08)70234-1

Petter, O. (2018, August 29). Going vegan is 'single biggest way' to reduce our impact on the planet, study finds. Retrieved from https://www.independent.co.uk/life-style/health-and-families/veganism-environmental-impact-planet-reduced-plant-based-diet-humans-study-a8378631.html.

Pietrocola, F., Malik, S. A., Mariño, G., Vacchelli, E., Senovilla, L., Chaba, K., … Kroemer, G. (2014). Coffee induces autophagy in vivo. Retrieved from https://www.ncbi.nlm.nih.gov/pmc/articles/PMC4111762/.

Poore, J., & Nemecek, T. (2018, June 1). Reducing food's environmental impacts through producers and consumers. Retrieved from https://science.sciencemag.org/content/360/6392/987.

Pradhan, R., Ashish, Peshin, A., Deshpande, M., Staughton, J., Vaidyanathan, V., ... Acharya, U. (2019, October 16). Cow Farts and Global Warming: Do Cows Contribute More to Global Warming? Retrieved from https://www.scienceabc.com/nature/cows-contribute-global-warming-cars.html.

Q&A on the carcinogenicity of the consumption of red meat and processed meat. (2016, May 17). Retrieved from https://www.who.int/features/qa/cancer-red-meat/en/.

Rizzo, N. S., Jaceldo-Siegl, K., Sabate, J., & Fraser, G. E. (2013). Nutrient Profiles of Vegetarian and Nonvegetarian Dietary Patterns. Journal of the Academy of Nutrition and Dietetics, 113(12), 1610–1619. doi: 10.1016/j.jand.2013.06.349

Robinson, J. (2013, May 25). Breeding the Nutrition Out of Our Food. Retrieved from https://www.nytimes.com/2013/05/26/opinion/sunday/breeding-the-nutrition-out-of-our-food.html?pagewanted=all&_r=0.

Santos-Longhurst, A. (2019, August 15). Type 2 Diabetes Statistics and Facts. Retrieved from https://www.healthline.com/health/type-2-diabetes/statistics#2.

Shalev, I., Entringer, S., Wadhwa, P. D., Wolkowitz, O. M., Puterman, E., Lin, J., & Epel, E. S. (2013, September). Stress and telomere biology: a lifespan perspective. Retrieved from https://www.ncbi.nlm.nih.gov/pubmed/23639252.

Skylark-Elizabeth, A. (2013, October 14). The Meat Industry Wastes Water. Retrieved from https://www.peta.org/blog/meat-industry-wastes-water/.

Smithers, R. (2018, November 1). Third of Britons have stopped or reduced eating meat - report. Retrieved from https://www.theguardian.com/business/2018/nov/01/third-of-britons-have-stopped-or-reduced-meat-eating-vegan-vegetarian-report.

Soliman, Sherry, Aronson, J., W., Barnard, & James, R. (2011, March 15). Analyzing Serum-Stimulated Prostate Cancer Cell Lines After Low-Fat, High-Fiber Diet and Exercise Intervention. Retrieved from https://www.hindawi.com/journals/ecam/2011/529053/.

Tiainen, A.-M. K., Männistö, S., Blomstedt, P. A., Moltchanova, E., Perälä, M.-M., Kaartinen, N. E., ... Eriksson, J. G. (2012, October 17). Leukocyte telomere length and its relation to food and nutrient intake in an elderly population. Retrieved from https://www.nature.com/articles/ejcn2012143.

Vanham, D., Comero, S., Gawlik, B. M., & Bidoglio, G. (2018, September 10). The water footprint of different diets within European sub-national geographical entities. Retrieved from https://www.nature.com/articles/s41893-018-0133-x.

Wang, B., Rong, X., Palladino, E. N., Wang, J., Fogelman, A. M., Martín, M. G., ... Tontonoz, P. (2018). Phospholipid Remodeling and Cholesterol Availability Regulate Intestinal Stemness and Tumorigenesis. Cell Stem Cell, 22(2). doi: 10.1016/j.stem.2017.12.017

Weroha, S. J., & Haluska, P. (2012, June). The insulin-like growth factor system in cancer. Retrieved from https://www.ncbi.nlm.nih.gov/pmc/articles/PMC3614012/.

Yue, W., Wang, J.-P., Li, Y., Fan, P., Liu, G., Zhang, N., ... Santen, R. (2010, October 15). Effects of estrogen on breast cancer development: Role of estrogen receptor independent mechanisms. Retrieved from https://www.ncbi.nlm.nih.gov/pmc/articles/PMC4775086/.

Printed in Great Britain
by Amazon

TARGET

COMPREHENSION

Chris Culshaw

OXFORD

OXFORD
UNIVERSITY PRESS

Great Clarendon Street, Oxford OX2 6DP

Oxford University Press is a department of the University of Oxford.
It furthers the University's objective of excellence in research,
scholarship, and education by publishing worldwide in

Oxford New York

Auckland Cape Town Dar es Salaam Hong Kong Karachi
Kuala Lumpur Madrid Melbourne Mexico City Nairobi
New Delhi Shanghai Taipei Toronto

With offices in

Argentina Austria Brazil Chile Czech Republic France
Greece Guatemala Hungary Italy Japan Poland Portugal
Singapore South Korea Switzerland Thailand Turkey
Ukraine Vietnam

Oxford is a registered trade mark of Oxford University Press
in the UK and in certain other countries

British Library Cataloguing in Publication Data

Data available

ISBN-13: 978 0 19 832015 9
ISBN-10: 0 19 832015 9

10 9 8 7 6 5 4

Designed and typeset by Mike Brain Graphic Design Limited, Oxford

Printed in Spain by Edelvives, Zaragoza

Contents

Drama

Non-fiction

To the Reader

'**Comprehension**' is just another word for 'understanding'. If we comprehend something we understand it; it makes sense. The aim of this book is to help you make sense of what you read.

In this book you will find poems, playscripts, adverts, newspaper articles, stories, instructions, etc. You can improve your comprehension of these kinds of materials by remembering this rule: **Different kinds of reading material require different kinds of reading.** This means we should vary the way we read, depending on the kind of material we are reading. For instance, we would read any instructions that came with a new music system very carefully. We would start at page one and try to follow them through, step-by-step. But when we read a magazine, we read whatever catches our eye first, and then skip around, until we've read it all.

Another thing to bear in mind is the difference between '**reading the lines**' and '**reading between the lines**'. For example, someone might have some sad news to pass on in a letter. This may be too painful to write about directly, so they may just hint at the news. We may therefore have to 'read between the lines' to know something is wrong. This comprehension skill is also useful when we read poetry and novels, which often have layers of meaning.

I hope you enjoy using this book as much as I have enjoyed putting it together. Sharpening your comprehension skills is well worth the effort. The more you understand, the more you can enjoy what you read. That's the way to make literacy work for you!

Chris Culshaw

Note to the teacher: The symbol **PF1** beside a writing activity indicates that this activity is supported by a photocopiable planning frame in the back of the Teacher's Book.

I was Haunted by the Internet

The only contact Elizabeth had with John was by computer ...

When Dad had the Internet added to our computer, it was brilliant. It took a bit of getting used to but, in the end, we all soon got the hang of it.

My mum loved it, because she could e-mail her sister in America – they were always swapping recipes and things. My dad's a doctor so he used it for work and helped me to use it, too.

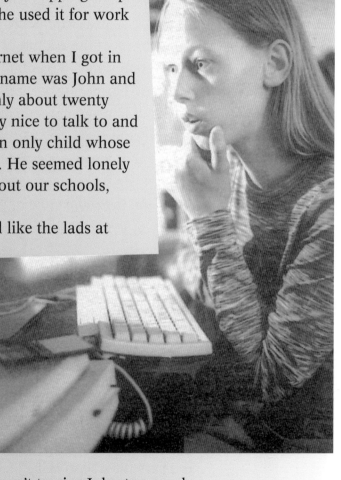

One night I was using the Internet when I got in touch with someone. He said his name was John and he lived in a village which was only about twenty miles from mine. He seemed really nice to talk to and he told me he was fourteen and an only child whose parents were a lot older than him. He seemed lonely and we passed on information about our schools, hobbies and pets.

He seemed grown up, not at all like the lads at school who just messed around all the time. John was different somehow. We arranged to talk again the following night and as he signed off I printed out our conversations to read over again later.

That night I kept thinking about John and the next morning over breakfast I told Mum all about him. Mum told me to be careful, she said that I wasn't to give John too much information because he might not be what he seemed. Although I thought he was my age, he could be much older and not the sort of person I should be getting friendly with.

I knew what Mum was getting at but I was sure John was worth getting to know.

FROM **SCARY STORIES** (PUBLISHED BY **SHOUT** MAGAZINE)

Understanding
1 What does Elizabeth's father do?
2 Which phrase tells you that Elizabeth lives in a village?
3 How far away from Elizabeth does John live?
4 In what way is John different to the boys at Elizabeth's school?
5 Why does Elizabeth's mother tell her to be careful? Suggest **one** thing Elizabeth should not do if she contacts John again.
6 The title of the story has more than one meaning. Write down **one** possible meaning. Compare this with your partner.

Extended Writing

PF 1 1 Write a short e-mail from Elizabeth to John in which she tells him a little bit about her school.

PF 2 2 In the extract, Elizabeth says John 'seemed lonely'. Write an e-mail from John to Elizabeth which contains some clues about his loneliness. Try to use some of the following words:

school   friends   hobby   shy   parents

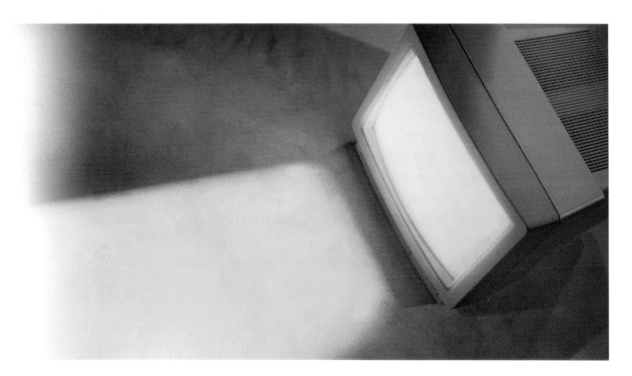

GLUED TO THE TELLY

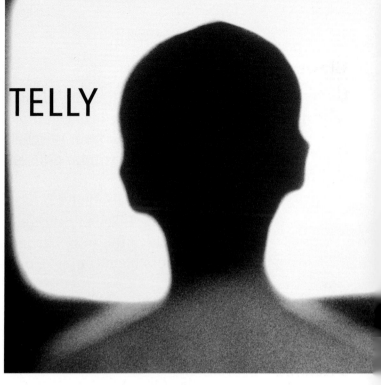

Herbert Hinckley loves the television. He doesn't go to school. He doesn't go out to play. He doesn't have any friends. He doesn't need them, because Herbert Hinckley loves the television.

He sits all day in his shabby red armchair, eating packets of crisps and drinking Coca Cola. His parents don't seem to mind. So long as Herbert is happy, they are happy. So Herbert just sits there, day in, day out, flicking between the channels, watching programme after mindless programme on a battered old television set.

If you ask Herbert what any of the programmes are about, he always replies, 'Cheese and Onion'. When Herbert watches the television, all he can think about is the flavour of his next packet of crisps.

The television set is as old as Herbert himself. His parents bought it for him on the day he was born. It has seen better days. The back is held on with rubber bands and garden string. The knobs on the front have long since dropped off and been replaced by lumps of half-chewed bubble gum. The screen has got a crack across it, that Herbert mended with Sellotape and sticking plaster.

'Would you like to sleep down here tonight, Herbert, as a treat?' said his mother one day.

'Cheese and Onion,' said Herbert …

An hour later, while Herbert slept, a silver grey cloud passed between the moon and Herbert's house. The sitting room was plunged into darkness. A streak of lightning cracked through the sky and struck the aerial that led directly into the back of Herbert's television. A switch clicked on. A faint humming sound grew from deep inside the belly of the machine. Then suddenly, BLIP! The television switched itself on. The little white dot that had been no bigger than a fingernail started to grow, getting larger and larger with every sleepy breath that Herbert took. It was as if Herbert and the television were breathing as one. The dot filled the screen and spread out into the room. It crept across the floor towards the sofa, edged over Herbert's pillow and onto his face. Herbert half opened one eye, but it was too late. The blinding light had completely surrounded him and suddenly, like a fisherman's net, it snatched him up and dragged him back through the television screen.

JAMIE RIX

Glossary .... **shabby:** worn-out, scruffy

mindless: without intelligence or thought

Understanding **1** What does Herbert think about as he watches television?

2 What kind of programmes does he watch?

3 In what ways is Herbert's television set like him?

4 How old do you think Herbert is? Use quotations from the extract to support your answer.

5 Why does the television switch itself on while Herbert is asleep?

6 What makes Herbert half open one eye?

Extended Writing .... **1** Copy and complete the table below.

Clue	What this tells us about Herbert
He doesn't go to school.	He may not be able to read, write or do maths. He may not know …
He doesn't go out to play.	He may not know very much about his street or town. He may not …
He doesn't have any friends.	
He watches TV all day.	
He only eats crisps.	

PF 3 **2** Describe what happens when Herbert appears in one of your favourite television programmes. Use information from the table in Question 1 (above). It will help you to decide what Herbert does. What does he say? How does he upset the programme?

THE WRECK OF THE ZANZIBAR

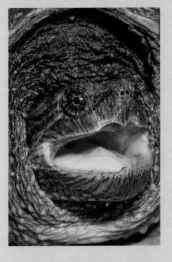

Today I found a turtle. I think it's called a leatherback turtle. I found one once before, but it was dead. This one had been washed up alive. Father had sent me down to collect driftwood on Rushy Bay. He said there'd be plenty about after a storm like that. He was right. I'd been there for half an hour or so heaping up the wood, before I noticed the turtle in the tideline of piled seaweed. I thought at first he was just a washed-up tree stump covered in seaweed. He was upside down on the sand. I pulled the seaweed off him. His eyes were open, unblinking. He was more dead than alive, I thought. He was massive, as long as this bed, and wider. He had a face like a two hundred year old man, wizened and wrinkled and with a gently-smiling mouth. I looked around, and there were more gulls gathering. They were silent, watching, waiting; and I knew well enough what they were waiting for. I pulled away more of the seaweed and saw that the gulls had been at him already. There was blood under his neck where the skin had been pecked. I had got there just in time.

MICHAEL MORPURGO

Glossary

driftwood: wood washed up on a beach by the sea

wizened: full of wrinkles

Understanding

1 Where is the narrator when she finds the turtle?
2 What is she doing there?
3 Why doesn't she see the turtle straight away?
4 List **three** facts about the turtle.
5 What does the narrator mean by 'I had got there just in time'?

Extended Writing

1 The narrator does not say how she feels when she goes to the beach, and sees the turtle and the gulls. We have to imagine her feelings. Copy and complete the table below. Try to find three or four words for each box. Use a thesaurus to help you.

What the narrator does	How she might be feeling
collects driftwood	hot, tired, bored
pulls the seaweed off the turtle	nervous, surprised …
looks at the turtle's face	
sees the gulls gathering	

2 Continue the story. Describe what the narrator does next. Also describe how she feels, using words from the table in Question 1 (above) and others.

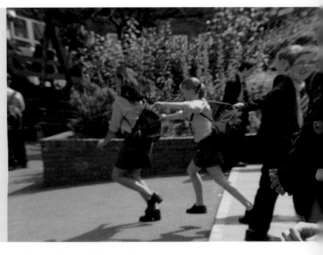

Annie's Game

Annie was talking to someone who wasn't there.

Jack looked across the school playground at his sister. She was nodding her head and smiling at the empty space next to her, waving her hands around as she talked. Jack wondered briefly why he was surprised. Nothing Annie did ought to surprise him any more. She was capable of anything, including having a conversation with thin air. Not that he cared what Annie was up to.

'Annie!' he called. 'Go and sit on the wall.'

Annie gave him a big smile.

'Can Sarah come with me?'

'What?' Jack turned to his sister.

'I said, "Can Sarah come with me?"'

'Sarah who?'

'Sarah Slade.' Annie pointed at the empty space next to her, a pleased look on her face.

'This is Sarah. She's my new friend. Say hello to Sarah, Jack.'

'There's no-one there,' Jack muttered.

'Yes, there is,' Annie retorted, unruffled. 'She's just invisible, that's all.'

'Of course she is,' said Jack. 'Silly me. I should have realized.'

'Don't be sarcastic, Jack.' Annie opened her eyes wide and gave him a superior stare. 'Sarah's a time-traveller, you know. She's come to visit me from the future.'

Jack resisted a desire to bang his head against the nearest brick wall. It was a feeling he often had when he was left alone with Annie.

'Look,' he said, unable to stand any more of what threatened to be yet another of Annie's endless games, 'go over there and sit on the wall. Have you got something to read?'

Annie pouted. 'I'd rather talk to Sarah.'

NARINDER DHAMI

Glossary

retorted: answered quickly

unruffled: calm

desire: a feeling of wanting something very much, a strong urge

pouted: pushed out their lips to show annoyance or sulking

Understanding

1 Where are Annie and Jack playing?

2 What is Annie doing that makes Jack think she is 'talking to thin air'?

3 What is Annie's 'new friend' called? Where is she from?

4 Who is the oldest – Annie or Jack? Use quotations from the extract to support your answer.

5 Annie's game makes Jack want to 'bang his head against the nearest brick wall'. What, in your own words, does this mean?

6 Which phrase tells you that Annie has played games like this before?

Extended Writing

1 What kind of relationship does Jack have with his sister? Write down what you think Jack thinks about Annie. Start like this:

Jack thinks Annie is …

Now write a similar sentence about Annie's feelings towards Jack. Start like this:

Annie thinks Jack is …

PF 4 2 Write a short monologue in which Annie talks to Sarah, her new friend, about her brother. Start like this:

That's my brother Jack over there. He doesn't believe in time-travel … Not like me …

Try to use some or all of the following words:

serious   fun   annoy   boring   older   trouble   friends

No Gun for Asmir

Asmir is living in Sarajevo with his mother, father, grandmother, and baby brother, Eldar. One day his world is turned upside down when the Serbian army attacks his home town. His father tells him they must leave.

Asmir put in their teddies, his best Lego and a bag of little farm animals, Eldar's cart and horse on wheels, a boat for the bath, some books, his coloured pencils, and drawing pad. His mother crammed T-shirts, jeans, shorts, pyjamas, shoes, and socks into a case.

Eldar was so restless that his mother slept beside him that night. So Asmir slept with his father. It was good to snuggle up with him. 'Why do we have to go away?' he asked. 'I don't want to leave you. Can't you come with us?'

'I wish I could,' his father said. 'But the war is getting worse every day. Yugoslavia has broken up. Serbia wants to take over Bosnia. That's why their army has invaded us.'

Invade. It was a crushing word. Asmir felt pinned down by it. As his friend had been by the falling wall.

His father went on. 'And women and children must have first chance to escape.'

Escape. A scary, running word. Almost worse than invade. His friend whose leg had been torn off by shrapnel couldn't run. He couldn't even walk. He couldn't escape.

'Why do we have to escape? Who are we escaping from?' Asmir's voice came out as a whisper in the dark.

'We're Muslim, Asmir. And *they* want to clean us out.'

'But we're clean already,' Asmir said, thinking of the washing dancing on the line, the gleaming copper cooking pots his grandmother loved to scour, the shining tiled floor, the crisp fresh clothes he put on each day. He stroked the smooth soft sheet. It was as soft as his grandmother's cheeks. And nobody could be cleaner than she was. 'Why do they want to clean us out? They're going about it in a very messy stupid way.'

He thought of the shattered glass, the piles of rubble, the splintered doors and sagging beams of houses in their own street, the proud trees in the playground blasted, split, stripped of their dancing leaves, dying.

'Who are *they*, anyway?'

Christobel Mattingley

Glossary

Bosnia: a small country in Eastern Europe between Hungary and Greece, part of former Yugoslavia

Serbia: a small country which borders on Bosnia, also part of former Yugoslavia

shrapnel: metal fragments from an exploding shell

Muslim: a person who follows the religious teachings of Muhammad

Understanding

1 In which city is Asmir living?

2 Why is Asmir's father staying behind?

3 What has happened to Asmir's friend?

4 **Paragraph 2** begins: 'Eldar was so restless ...' Use a dictionary or thesaurus to find **three** words that the author could have used instead of 'restless'.

5 Look up the meaning of the following words:

angry   anxious   confused.

Which word best describes how Asmir feels about leaving his home? Choose **one** short quotation from the extract to support your answer.

Extended Writing

Asmir and his family leave their home that night. The streets are deserted. There are no street lights but there is a full moon. Write two short paragraphs about Asmir's escape.

Paragraph 1   Describe what Asmir sees as he leaves his house and walks down his street past the playground. You could begin like this:

Asmir carried his baby brother, Eldar, on his back. His mother was carrying a heavy suitcase. In the case were ...

Paragraph 2   Describe what Asmir feels as he leaves his home town. Try to link the way he feels with the smashed buildings and trees and the way they look in the moonlight. You could begin like this:

The bright moonlight shone down on the smashed houses. They looked as if they were made of ice. Asmir shivered.

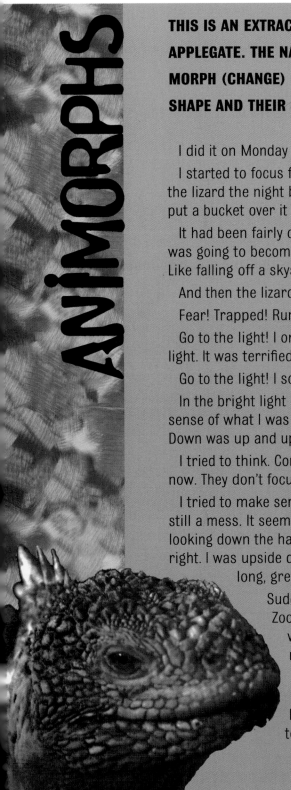

ANIMORPHS

THIS IS AN EXTRACT FROM ANIMORPHS 1: THE INVASION BY K. A. APPLEGATE. THE NARRATOR, JAKE, HAS A STRANGE POWER. HE CAN MORPH (CHANGE) INTO DIFFERENT ANIMALS. HE TAKES ON THEIR SHAPE AND THEIR SENSES.

I did it on Monday morning in my locker at school. I turned into a lizard.

I started to focus for the morphing. I remembered the way we had caught the lizard the night before last. We'd spotted it with a torch, and Cassie had put a bucket over it so it couldn't get away.

It had been fairly creepy, just touching it to acquire its DNA pattern. Now I was going to become it. Things began to happen very fast. It was like falling. Like falling off a skyscraper and taking for ever to hit the ground.

And then the lizard brain kicked in.

Fear! Trapped! Run! Run! Rruunrunrun!

Go to the light! I ordered my new body. But the body was afraid of the light. It was terrified.

Go to the light! I screamed inside my head. And suddenly I was there.

In the bright light I realized how bad the lizard eyes were. I couldn't make sense of what I was seeing. Everything was shattered and twisted around. Down was up and up was down.

I tried to think. Come on, Jake. You have eyes on the side of your head now. They don't focus together. They see different things. Deal with it.

I tried to make sense of the pictures, using this knowledge, but they were still a mess. It seemed to take me for ever to figure it out. One eye was looking down the hall to the left. The other was looking down the hall to the right. I was upside down, gripping the side of the locker, which was like a long, grey field that wouldn't end.

Suddenly I was off and running. Straight down the wall. Zoom! Then on level floor. Zoom! The ground flew past. It was like being strapped on to a crazy, out-of-control missile.

Then my lizard brain sensed the spider. It was a strange thing, like I wasn't sure if I saw the spider, or heard it, or smelled it, or tasted it on my flicking lizard tongue, or just suddenly knew it was there.

K. A. APPLEGATE

Glossary ....

morphing: changing shape

acquire: obtain, take on

DNA pattern: information about the biological make-up of a living thing

Understanding

1 When and where does Jake morph into a lizard?

2 Why did Jake need to touch the lizard?

3 Which sentence tells you that morphing happens quickly?

4 How is a lizard's vision different from human sight?

5 Jake feels as if he is 'strapped on to a crazy, out-of-control missile'. Why?

6 What senses are mentioned in the last paragraph? What does the spider incident tell you about a lizard's senses and how they are different from human senses?

Extended Writing ....

1 Make a list of phrases from the extract which suggest Jake found morphing a frightening thing to do. Begin like this:

'Like falling off a skyscraper'

'Fear! Trapped! Run!'

PF5 **2** Write the next part of the story in which Jake morphs into another animal and explores a place that you know well (e.g. a room in your school, your bedroom, your local supermarket or park). Write two paragraphs.

Paragraph 1 Describe how Jake morphs. Use words and phrases from Question 1 (above) to show how he feels as this happens.

Paragraph 2 Describe what Jake sees through the animal's eyes. Remember, even the most ordinary things will seem strange, even frightening.

Peter Hawkins

Every night, at the same time, our stepfather's keys rattled at the front door. Boots brushed and scraped on the doormat. In came Peter Hawkins, a red face sticking out of wide blue overalls smeared with car grease. Before tea, our stepfather scrubbed the oil from his face and hands at the kitchen sink. He combed his black hair flat against his skull and flicked the dandruff from his shoulders. Under the soapy scent, we caught faint whiffs of petroleum when he smacked our cheeks with kisses.

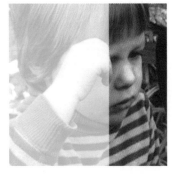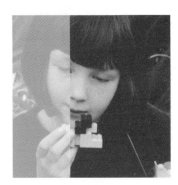

Tea was ketchup with mashed potato and things out of tins, baked beans or spaghetti. We ate it without a word while our stepfather sat chomping and staring over our heads at the telly. After tea, our mother washed the dishes, washed our faces and changed into a stiff green dress that zipped up the front. Then she folded into her car – a battered blue Princess whose patches of rust she was forever daubing with metallic paint – and drove off to look after dying people until dawn. She worked the night shift at Manchester City Council Home for Geriatrics.

'It's at night that they pop their clogs, that's the worst part,' she told Auntie Livia, describing the toothless corpses that she lifted from their still-warm beds. 'Their faces are smiling – sort of floating up – but their legs feel like lead.'

While she swept corridors and bathed worn-out brows, our stepfather was left with my sisters and me. Lulled by soap operas, his eyelids drooped over a warm can of beer. Sarah slept cradled on his dozing belly, calmly rising and falling, while Laurie and I played in silence behind the dining table.

We were allowed to play with Lego, but only if we pressed the bricks together without any clicking sounds. Our heads were crammed with Lego helicopters and dinosaurs, but we put all our bricks into building ships to please our stepfather. He slumped back on the settee while the television's light flickered electric over his features, now blue, now red.

FROM *ONCE IN A HOUSE ON FIRE* BY ANDREA ASHWORTH

Glossary

whiffs: slight smells

petroleum: petrol

chomping: eating noisily

Princess: an Austin Princess, a make of car

daubing: painting clumsily

Geriatrics: old people too ill to care for themselves

pop their clogs: slang for 'die'

corpses: dead bodies

lulled: sent to sleep (gently)

features: parts of the face, e.g. eyes, nose, mouth

Understanding

1 Who is Peter Hawkins?

2 What is his job? What is the narrator's mother's job?

3 Why does Peter fall asleep in front of the television?

4 What do the narrator and Laurie make from Lego? Suggest **one** reason why they do this.

5 How old do you think Sarah is? Support your answer with a quotation from the extract.

6 How does Peter Hawkins feel about his stepchildren? Give reasons for your answer.

7 The first sentence: 'Every night, at the same time …' tells you that Peter likes to be punctual, and always sticks to a regular routine. Pick another sentence from the first paragraph and say what this tells you about Peter's character.

Extended Writing

1 List all the information in the extract about the narrator's mother and the job she does. Begin like this:

She goes to work in an old battered car.

She works at night, in an old people's home.

2 Use the information from Question 1 (above) to write a short pen portrait of the narrator's mother. You will need to invent some details, such as her age, height, hair colour, etc. But you will be able to work out quite a bit about her character from the extract, as you did with Peter (see Question 7, above).

Fiction

The Present

This is an extract from *Kit's Wilderness* by David Almond. It is Christmas Day. Just as dawn is breaking, Kit's grandfather comes to his room. He tells Kit he has a present for him and leads him into his own bedroom.

'This is for you,' he said.

I looked around for a present, saw his souvenirs on the shelves, fossils and little carvings, ancient photographs of his pit mates, the wardrobe with the cuff of a white shirt caught in the door, slippers on the floor, the wedding photograph, his bed with the impression of his frail body on it.

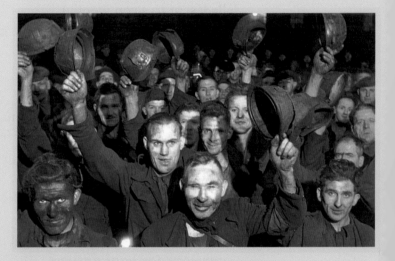

'What is?' I said.

He grinned. 'Everything is. Everything is yours.'

I didn't know what to say.

'Have to hang on to a few of the things a while longer,' he said. 'But afterwards they come to you, to keep or chuck as you wish. Everything.'

I gazed around the room again as the light grew and shone in upon these gifts. His eyes were shining.

'What I'd like to give you most of all is what's inside. The tales and memories and dreams that keep the world alive.' He squeezed my arm.

I touched the photographs, the fossil tree, the shirt cuff, felt how they burned with Grandpa's life, and with those tales and memories and dreams.

'OK?' he whispered.

'Yes.' I put my arms around him, held him as we'd held each other in the darkest tunnels of our dreams. 'Thank you, Grandpa.'

He sighed.

'One day,' he whispered. 'I won't be here any more. You know that, Kit. But I'll live on inside you and then inside your own children and grandchildren. We'll go on forever, you and me and all the ones that's gone and all the ones that's still to come.'

And the light intensified around us, bringing Grandpa's final Christmas Day.

Glossary

souvenirs: things you keep to remind you of people or places
pit mates: fellow workers in a mine
impression: a mark pressed into something (such as a footprint in sand)
frail: fragile, not strong
intensified: grew stronger, brighter

Understanding

1 Kit's grandfather was once a coal miner. Which object in his room tells you this?

2 Pick another object that you think has special memories for the old man and say why.

3 When Kit touches the objects, how do they feel? Say, in your own words, what this tells you about the old man's life.

4 What did Kit's grandfather mean by 'We'll go on forever, you and me'?

5 What does the last sentence of the extract tell you about the old man?

6 What does the extract tell you about the character of Kit and his relationship with his grandfather? Use quotations from the extract to support your answer.

Extended Writing

1 Make a list of **five** or **six** objects which you treasure. Say how you came to own each object and why it has a special meaning for you.

2 Imagine that these objects are discovered by a member of your family long after you are dead. Each would be a small clue to your life and your personality. What conclusions would they come to about you? Write a sentence like this about each object:

This object will tell them that I ...

Wilderness House

This is an extract from **The House of Wings** by Betsy Byars. Sammy's parents have gone to Detroit to find work. Sammy wants to go with them, but is made to stay with his grandfather, on his farm. Sammy runs away, to try to find his parents. His grandfather runs after him.

Sammy crouched in the metal culvert that ran beneath the highway. His head was bent forward over his dusty knees. His shoulders were hunched, his eyes shut. He was listening.

At first there was only the sound of his own ragged breathing and the hum of cars on the highway above. Then he heard it.

'Boy!'

Sammy's head snapped up. He stared at the circle of light at the end of the culvert. He waited. His face was dusty and, beneath the dust, red. Tears had washed the dust away in streaks down the sides of his cheeks. He had cried so hard that he had got the hiccups.

'Boy, where are you?' his grandfather called. 'Boy!'

Sammy did not answer. He remained bent over in the position of a runner about to start a race. One hand, still wet with tears, was braced on his knee; the other hung at his side. His fingers nervously pinched up the pale sand in the bottom of the culvert and released it.

'Boy, are you in that pipe? You hear me?' His grandfather's voice was louder and Sammy knew he was close, probably climbing the bank right now. 'Do you hear me?'

Sammy ran in a crouch through the pipe. He came out the other side in the grass divide between the highways and waited. He was bent over in a knot. He hiccuped loudly.

Someone threw an empty Fresca can from one of the passing cars, and it rolled down the bank. Sammy raised his head. He saw the cars flashing by and the sky beyond, which was the bright blue of cornflowers.

He did not move. After a moment he leaned over and glanced through the pipe. At that exact moment his grandfather looked through the pipe on the other side and they saw each other. It was a strange sensation. It was as if they were the only two people in the world, staring at each other through the centre of the earth.

Glossary

Detroit: a city in Michigan, USA
culvert: drainpipe passing under a road or railway
highway: main road or route
Fresca: a kind of soft drink
sensation: feeling

Understanding

1 Where is Sammy hiding?
2 What sounds does he hear as he crouches in his hiding place?
3 How does Sammy know that his grandfather is getting closer?
4 Where is Sammy when he comes out of the other end of the pipe?
5 What came rolling down the bank next to Sammy?
6 Why doesn't Sammy answer his grandfather's calls?

Extended Writing

1 Read the extract again and look for any clues that might tell you about the relationship between Sammy and his grandfather. Begin like this:

His grandfather calls him 'Boy', not Sammy. This is a rather cold way for him to speak to Sammy.

Sammy has been crying. He may have had an argument with his grandfather.

PF 6 **2** When Sammy comes face to face with his grandfather, they talk about why the boy ran away. Write down what they say to each other. Show what kind of a relationship they have through what they say and how they say it. Set it out like a playscript. You could begin like this:

Grandfather: (Angrily) Are you deaf, Boy? Didn't you hear me shouting?

Sammy: (In a whisper) I heard.

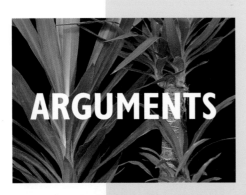

ARGUMENTS

This is an extract from *Meteorite Spoon* by Philip Ridley. Filly and Fergal's parents, Mr and Mrs Thunder, are always arguing. Filly and Fergal share a bedroom. One morning Filly is awakened by her brother talking in his sleep.

'Arguments, Sis!'

Filly's eyes clicked open.

'Arguments, Sis!'

Filly leaned over the edge of her top bunk and looked at Fergal, who was asleep in the bottom one.

He was thrashing about in the throes of a nightmare, twisting and turning, entangling himself in the sheets.

Immediately, Filly jumped out of bed and tried to wake him.

'Buck up, Brov!' she said, shaking his shoulder. 'It's only a nightmare!'

Whenever Fergal was particularly upset by the arguments, he had nightmares. Filly guessed it was yesterday's 'The Argument that Broke the Washing-machine' that had triggered this one. After all, it did last for seven hours and thirty-two minutes and seventeen seconds, and Filly and Fergal had to sit in their bedroom, listening, without anything to eat or drink. They'd been faint with hunger and thirst by the time it was all over.

'Arguments, Sis!'

'Crikey, Brov, please buck up.'

Filly was getting very worried about Fergal. Once before, almost three months ago now (after 'The Argument that Broke the Yucca Plant'), Fergal had got himself into such a state that he'd run down into the cellar and cried and cried for hours and hours.

There was nothing Filly could do to stop him. She told him to 'buck up' and things like that, but it did no good. Fergal just sobbed and sobbed, until his jumper got so wet Filly was afraid it might shrink.

'Come back upstairs, Brov,' she had said.

'Nope, Sis,' Fergal had replied tearfully.

'Why not, Brov?'

'Arguments, Sis.'

'So how long are you going to stay down here, Brov?'

'For ever, Sis.'

But, of course, he didn't.

And, for a while, it seemed as if he was coping.

But now the nightmares were back!

Crikey, thought Filly, I hope poor Brov doesn't start crying again. His jumper will shrink for sure next time.

Filly grabbed hold of Fergal's shoulders and shook him so hard a bed-spring went 'TWANG'!

It was the twanging rather than the shaking that woke him.

Glossary

thrashing: moving violently
in the throes of: struggling with (the nightmare)
buck up: slang for 'cheer up'
yucca plant: plant with spiky leaves
coping: managing

Understanding

1 How does Filly know Fergal is having a nightmare?
2 What does Filly think has triggered her brother's nightmare?
3 Where does Fergal run to hide, after the Yucca plant argument?
4 When did their parents argue about the washing-machine? How long did this argument last?
5 Which phrases tell you that Fergal is in a very deep sleep?
6 Why, in your own words, is Filly 'very worried about Fergal'?

Extended Writing

1 Filly keeps a record of all her parents' arguments. She writes them down in a big black book which she calls 'The Book of Arguments'. She writes down what they argue about, what gets broken and how long each argument lasts.

Write an entry for Filly's black book. Describe how the argument started, what it was about and how long it lasted. Remember, Filly writes about all her parents' arguments in a light-hearted way. Try to do the same.

2 Filly treats the arguments like some kind of game. She thinks this will help Fergal and stop him getting so upset. What do you think? Write a paragraph giving your views on how Filly is trying to help her brother. Suggest other ways she might try to help Fergal. Begin like this:

I think Filly's 'Book of Arguments' is a good/bad/stupid/clever idea because ...

Try to use the following words:

Fergal   upset   help   understand   better   worse

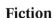

WAR HORSE

Joey, the narrator, is a cavalry horse fighting with the British army, in France, during the First World War. Topthorn, another horse, is fighting alongside Joey as they charge a line of German trenches. Trooper Warren is Joey's rider.

Trooper Warren prayed aloud as he rode, but his prayers turned soon to curses as he saw the carnage around him. Only a few horses reached the wire and Topthorn and I were amongst them. There were indeed a few holes blasted through the wire by our bombardment so that some of us could find a way through; and we came at last upon the first line of enemy trenches, but they were empty. The firing came now from higher up in amongst the trees; and so the squadron, or what was left of it, regrouped and galloped up into the wood, only to be met by a line of hidden wire in amongst

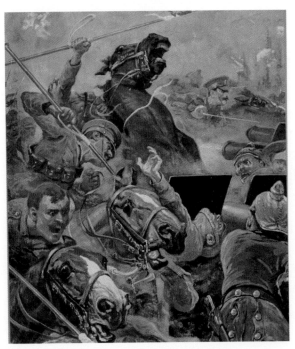

the trees. Some of the horses ran into the wire before they could be stopped, and stuck there, their riders trying feverishly to extract them. I saw one trooper dismount deliberately once he saw his horse was caught. He pulled out his rifle and shot his mount before falling dead himself on the wire. I could see at once that there was no way through, that the only way was to jump the wire and when I saw Topthorn and Captain Stewart leap over where the wire was lowest, I followed them and we found ourselves at last in amongst the enemy. From behind every tree, from trenches all around it seemed, they ran forward in their piked helmets to counter-attack. They rushed past us, ignoring us until we found ourselves surrounded by an entire company of soldiers, their rifles pointing up at us.

The crump of shelling and the spitting of rifle-fire had suddenly stopped. I looked around me for the rest of the squadron, to discover that we were alone. Behind us the riderless horses, all that was left of a proud cavalry squadron, galloped back towards our trenches, and the hillside below was strewn with the dead and dying.

'Throw down your sword, Trooper,' said Captain Stewart, bending in his saddle and dropping his sword to the ground. 'There's been enough useless slaughter today. No sense in adding to it.'

MICHAEL MORPURGO

Glossary

trooper: a soldier who fights on horseback

carnage: mass killing

bombardment: an attack by shells from heavy guns

squadron: a group, or unit, of soldiers

feverishly: frantically, in a desperate way

extract: set free

piked helmets: German helmets with a spike on top

counter-attack: fight back

crump of shelling: the dull thud of shell-fire

slaughter: killing

Understanding

1 Who is Trooper Warren?

2 Why are Joey and Topthorn able to find a way through the wire?

3 What do they see at the first line of enemy trenches?

4 Who is Captain Stewart?

5 What happens to many of the horses as they gallop into the wood?

6 Why, in your own words, does Captain Stewart tell Trooper Warren to stop fighting? Try to think of **two** reasons for his decision.

Extended Writing

1 Read through the extract again. Pick out as many phrases as you can that tell you the fight is a desperate struggle. Begin like this:

'his prayers turned soon to curses'

'he saw the carnage around him'

'Only a few horses reached the wire'

PF 7 **2** Trooper Warren becomes a prisoner of war. He writes a letter home to his parents. He describes how he was captured. He is proud of the men and their horses. But he feels very sad about his dead and wounded companions. Write the letter, using words and phrases from Question 1 (above). Think about who the letter is sent to. How will this affect what Trooper Warren says in his letter?

Ears, Eyes, Legs, and Arms

Once, long ago, the different parts of the body weren't all together but went about the world on their own. The ears, the eyes, the legs, and the arms all went about their business, doing what they had to do – ears one way, eyes the other, legs off over there, arms over the other way.

One day though, they decided to go out hunting together. The ears, eyes, legs, and arms marched off to the forest.

They walked for seven days before they got there but just as they were getting near, the ears called out, 'Shh, listen! I can hear something.'

Immediately the eyes started to search among the trees, and then suddenly they called out, 'There! Look! An antelope! Over there …'

The legs set off to chase it, followed closely by the arms. As the legs caught up with the antelope, the arms reached out and killed it.

After a while, the ears and the eyes caught up with their friends.

'What do you want?' said the arms. 'The antelope's ours, we caught it. Shove off.'

'No, come off it,' said the legs. 'You would never have been able to grab it if it wasn't for us being fast enough to catch up with it.'

'Never mind that,' said the eyes. 'We reckon the antelope's ours, because we were the ones who saw it. You wouldn't have known where to go if it wasn't for us.'

'All right, all right,' said the ears. 'Who got the whole thing going? Us, of course. We heard the antelope, didn't we? You'd all be sitting around back there if it wasn't for us hearing it move.'

This story, from Mali in Africa, was collected by Ced Hesse and told to him by Mamadou Karambe.

(continued on page 30)

Glossary   **antelope:** an animal like a deer

Understanding **1** Why do the body parts go into the forest?
2 Which body part first notices the antelope?
3 Which body part kills the antelope?

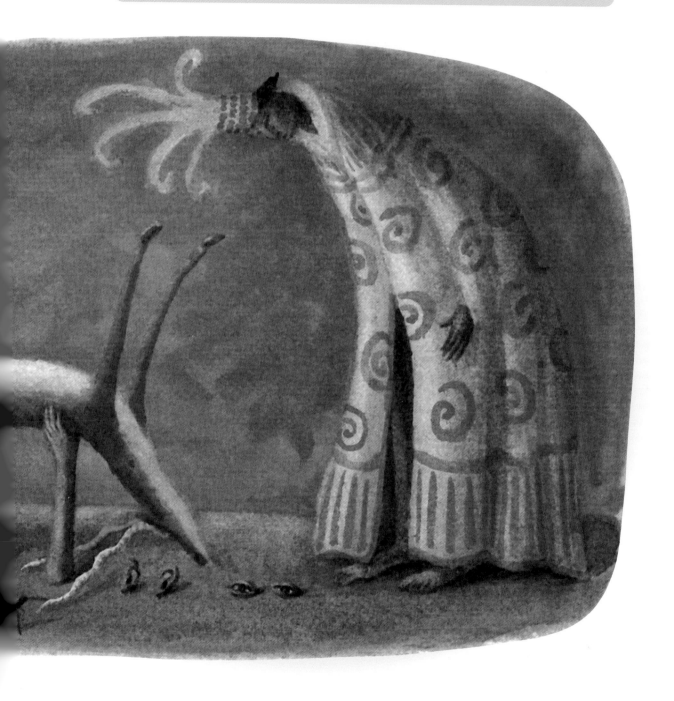

Just then a mosquito came by.

'What's the row about? What's all the fuss about?'

They told it the story.

'Hmm,' said the mosquito, 'this is a tricky one. Very tricky. But listen, there's a wise old chief not far from here – why not take the problem to him?'

Off went the four friends to the wise old chief, with the arms carrying the antelope.

The chief listened to the story and then ordered the antelope to be cooked. When it was brought to him, he sat down and started eating. He didn't stop till he had finished every last bit. And not once did he ask the four friends to have some.

Then the chief spoke. 'I listened to your story and decided that I would punish all of you for being so mean and selfish. First I punished you by eating all of the antelope without sharing any of it with you. Now I am going to punish you all once more, by joining you together so that something like this never happens again.'

And he did.

The parts of the body were furious with the chief for doing this, but they were even angrier with the mosquito for bringing them to see the chief. And that's why whenever the ears hear the whine of a mosquito, the eyes search for it and the arms try and slap it. If, as often happens, the mosquito still whines, even after the arms have slapped and smacked all over the place, the legs join in the hunt.

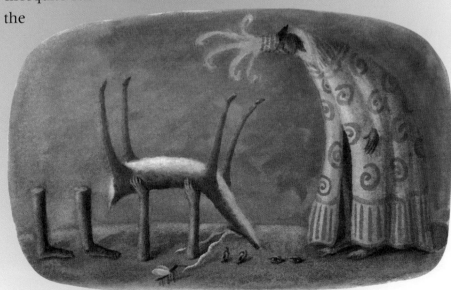

Glossary .... **mosquito:** small gnat (fly) that sucks blood

whine: the high-pitched buzz of a small insect

Understanding **4** Why does the mosquito take the body parts to the chief?

5 What does the chief do **before** he speaks to the body parts?

6 Why, in your own words, does the chief punish them?

7 What is the moral of the story? Is it an important moral? Give reasons for your answer.

Extended Writing .... **1** Copy and complete this table, which shows how each body part might help when cooking a meal.

Ears	can hear kettle/pan boil	can hear cooker timer ping
Eyes	can see vegetables are…	can see …
Legs		
Arms		

2 Use the table in Question 1 (above) to write a dialogue between two different body parts who argue about who is the most important, when they cook a special meal. You could start like this:

Arms: I'm the most important!

Eyes: Why?

Arms: Because I carried all the food home from the shop.

Eyes: You would never have found the shop without me.

Godzilla

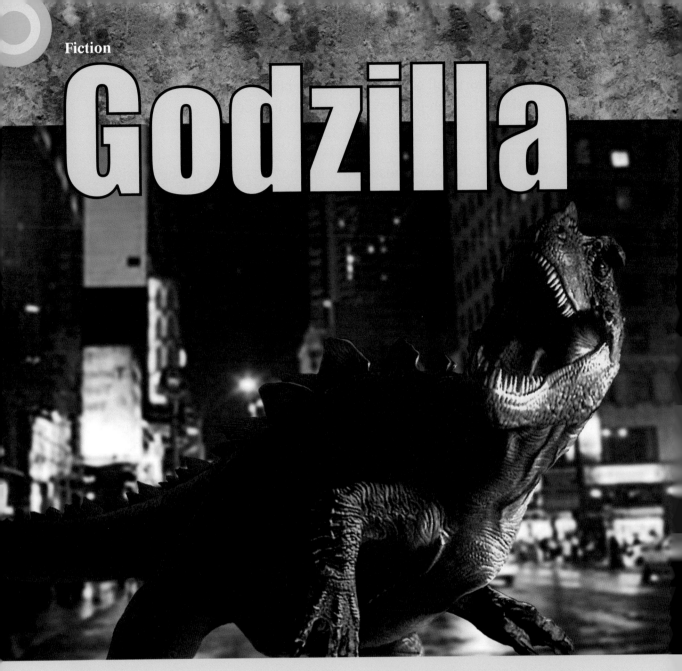

THE OLD TRAMP was carrying a battered fishing rod. Turning his greasy collar up against the rain, he shuffled past the loading-docks and busy stalls of New York City's Fulton Fish Market.

The pavement was oily and glistening with scales. Not even the driving rain could wash away the stench of fish.

The tramp stopped to rest under the FDR Drive.

'Gonna get yourself some lunch?' a man sitting on a filthy bare mattress, his back against one of the highway's girders, called out to him. 'Gonna catch one of them delicious East River fish?'

In the shadowy darkness, several other men sniggered and laughed.

'You never know,' the old tramp answered. 'Sometimes you get lucky.'

He left the shelter of the overpass and

walked out on to the pier. At the furthest edge of the dock he sat down and cast his line into the murky water.

Within seconds, the floating lure bobbed. The pole bent. The old man smiled to himself.

Suddenly the water began to churn. Something enormous started to rise out of the scummy river.

The old man's red-rimmed eyes bulged. He swallowed hard and scrambled to his feet as the huge back fins of a tremendous reptile burst out of the river.

The tramp dropped his rod and took off, running. The dock behind him was ripped apart as an awesome force came up from beneath it.

Slipping and sliding in the rain, the tramp skidded under the Drive. Shivering with fear, he hid behind a steel girder.

The creature rose, sending a tidal wave of water crashing down on the elevated highway, bending the steel girder like a paperclip.

(continued on page 34)

Glossary

scales: thin flakes of skin on a fish

stench: a very bad smell

FDR Drive: fly-over named after American president, Franklin D. Roosevelt

girders: thick metal beams holding up part of a bridge or building

overpass: a roadway carrying traffic over another roadway (a fly-over)

murky: dark, dirty

lure: float used to attract fish

churn: swirl, move in a quick or violent way

scummy: having a layer of dirt floating on its surface

awesome: fearful, frightening

elevated: raised up, above the ground

highway: main road or route

Understanding

1 Where is the old tramp going and why is he going there?
2 Where are the other men sheltering?
3 One of the men asks the tramp if he is going to catch 'one of them delicious East River fish'. Why does he use the word 'delicious'?
4 What happens as the tramp is running along the dock?
5 Where does the tramp hide?
6 What happens as the creature comes up out of the water? What does this tell us about the size of the creature?

Godzilla

A car was washed over the guardrail. A yellow cab landed on top of it, crushing its bonnet. Screams erupted. The battered driver crawled out of the smashed taxi and was sucked into the river as the immense wave retreated.

Overhead, on the Drive, cars and trucks crashed and scraped against one another. Horns began to blare. People shrieked.

An enormous foot with massive claws stepped over the highway, shattering the pavement.

Cars swerved to get out of the way. A boat that had been tossed up from the river, crashed down, severing the Drive. A van collided with the boat.

In one immense motion, an impossibly huge tail with a ridge of razor-sharp scales dragged across the Drive, sweeping the road clear of wreckage.

The earth shook as the creature moved inland towards the fish market.

Suddenly a truck was lifted into the air, and a shower of crushed ice and hulking fish rained down on the street.

H.B. GILMOUR

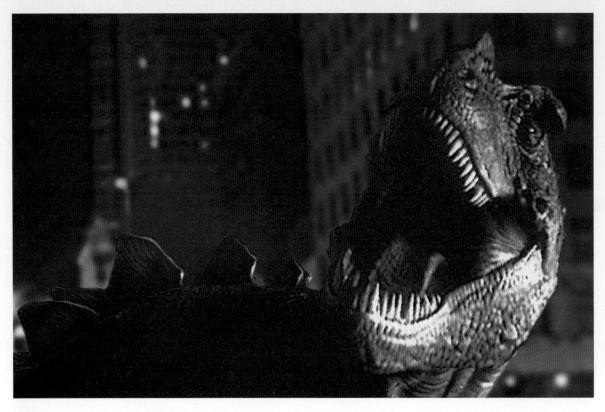

Glossary

guardrail: a safety rail, to stop traffic driving off the overpass
cab: taxi
immense: huge
blare: make a loud blast of noise
severing: cutting in two
motion: movement
hulking: large, heavy

Understanding

7 Pick out **one** phrase or sentence which tells you the creature is very strong.

8 What, in your own words, happens to the taxi driver?

9 What do you think happens to the other men who were sheltering near the dock? Give a reason for your answer.

Extended Writing

1 Read the extract again. Imagine you are the tramp. Make a list of all the sounds you would hear. Begin like this:

the voices of men and women at the fish market

the hiss of the rain on the dock

the roar of traffic on FDR Drive (the overpass)

PF 8 **2** Write the next part of the story. The creature, Godzilla, moves into the city. Think about where it strikes next – the 'setting'. It could be a cinema, a supermarket, a school. Write three short paragraphs. Think carefully about the sounds you would hear.
Paragraph 1 Describe the setting before the creature strikes.
Paragraph 2 Describe what happens when it strikes.
Paragraph 3 Describe the scene after the creature has moved on.

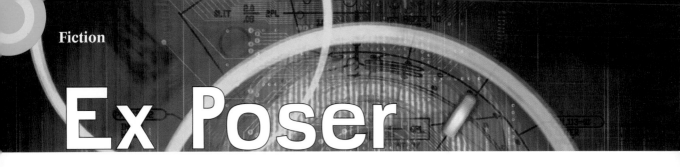

Fiction

Ex Poser

There are two rich kids in our form. Sandra Morris and Ben Fox. They are both snobs. They think they are too good for the rest of us. Their parents have big cars and big houses. Both of them are quiet. They keep to themselves. I guess they don't want to mix with the ruffians like me.

Ben Fox always wears expensive gym shoes and the latest fashions. He thinks he is good-looking with his blue eyes and blonde hair. He is a real poser.

Sandra Morris is the same. And she knows it. Blue eyes and blonde hair too. Skin like silk. Why do some kids get the best of everything?

Me, I landed pimples. I've used everything I can on them. But still they bud and grow and burst. Just when you don't want them to. It's not fair.

Anyway, today I have the chance to even things up. Boffin is bringing along his latest invention – a lie detector. Sandra Morris is the victim. She agreed to try it out because everyone knows that she would never tell a lie. What she doesn't know is that Boffin and I are going to ask her some very embarrassing questions.

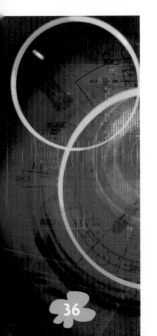

Boffin is a brain. His inventions always work. He is smarter than the teachers. Everyone knows that. And now he has brought along his latest effort. A lie detector.

He tapes two wires to Sandra's arm. 'It doesn't hurt,' he says. 'But it is deadly accurate.' He switches on the machine and a little needle swings into the middle of the dial. 'Here's a trial question,' he says. 'Are you a girl?'

Sandra nods.

'You have to say yes or no,' he says.

'Yes,' replies Sandra. The needle swings over to TRUTH. Maybe this thing really works. Boffin gives a big grin.

'This time tell a lie,' says Boffin. 'Are you a girl?' he asks again.

Sandra smiles with that lovely smile of hers. 'No,' she says. A little laugh goes up but then all the kids in the room gasp. The needle points to LIE. This lie detector is a terrific invention.

'Okay,' says Boffin. 'You only have seven questions, David. The batteries will go flat after another seven questions.' He sits down behind his machine and twiddles the knobs.

This is going to be fun. I am going to find out a little bit about Sandra Morris and Ben Fox. It's going to be very interesting. Very interesting indeed.

I ask my first question. 'Have you ever kissed Ben Fox?'

Sandra goes red. Ben Fox goes red. I have got them this time. I am sure they have something going between them. I will expose them.

'No,' says Sandra. Everyone cranes their neck to see what the lie detector says. The needle points to TRUTH.

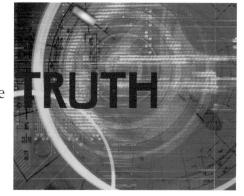

(continued on page 38)

Glossary

ruffians: badly behaved people, yobs
pimples: spots
lie detector: a machine that shows if someone is lying
twiddles: twists something quickly to and fro
crane their neck: stretch their necks in an effort to see

Understanding

1 Why does the narrator dislike Sandra and Ben?
2 In what ways do Ben and Sandra look alike?
3 Which phrase in the fifth paragraph tells you that the lie detector isn't the only thing Boffin has invented?
4 How many questions can David (the narrator) ask?
5 What is the first question he asks? Why does he ask this?

Fiction

This is not what I expected. And I only have six questions left. I can't let her off the hook. I am going to expose them both.

'Have you ever held his hand?'

Again she says, 'No.' And the needle says TRUTH. I am starting to feel guilty. Why am I doing this?

I try another tack. 'Are you in love?' I ask.

A red flush starts to creep up her neck. I am feeling really mean now. Fox is blushing like a sunset.

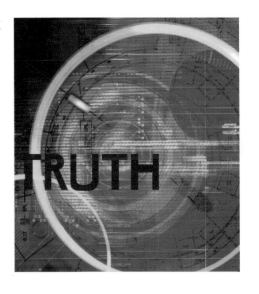

'Yes,' she says. The needle points to TRUTH.

I shouldn't have let the kids talk me into doing this. I decide to put Sandra and Ben out of their agony. I won't actually name him. I'll spare her that. 'Is he in this room?' I say.

She looks at the red Ben Fox. 'Yes,' she says. The needle points to TRUTH.

'Does he have blue eyes?' I ask.

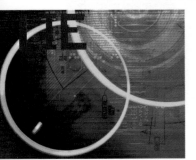

'No,' she says.

'Brown?' I say.

'No,' she says again.

I don't know what to say next. I look at each kid in the class very carefully. Ben Fox has blue eyes. I was sure that she loved him.

'This thing doesn't work,' I say to Boffin. 'I can't see one kid who doesn't have either blue eyes or brown eyes.'

'We can,' says Boffin. They are all looking at me.

I can feel my face turning red now. I wish I could sink through the floor but I get on with my last question. 'Is he an idiot?' I ask.

Sandra is very embarrassed. 'Yes,' she says in a voice that is softer than a whisper. 'And he has green eyes.'

FROM *UNMENTIONABLE* BY PAUL JENNINGS

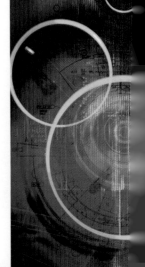

Glossary

off the hook: escape (as a fish might get 'off' the hook)
expose: to reveal the hidden truth about someone or something
flush: blush
agony: misery, pain, an uncomfortable situation

Understanding

6 What, in your own words, does David mean when he decides to 'put Sandra and Ben out of their agony'?

7 What colour are David's eyes? Give a reason for your answer.

8 When Sandra speaks, her voice is 'softer than a whisper'. What does this tell you about her feelings for David?

Extended Writing

1 Read the extract again and pick out all the information about the lie detector and how it works. Begin like this:

It is Boffin's latest invention.
Boffin's inventions always work.
It does not hurt.

PF 9 **2** Write another story about Boffin and his lie detector in which he helps Ben Fox find his missing trainers. Use information about the machine, from Question 1 (above). You could begin your story like this:

'Oh no!' cried Ben, when he opened his bag. 'They've gone!'

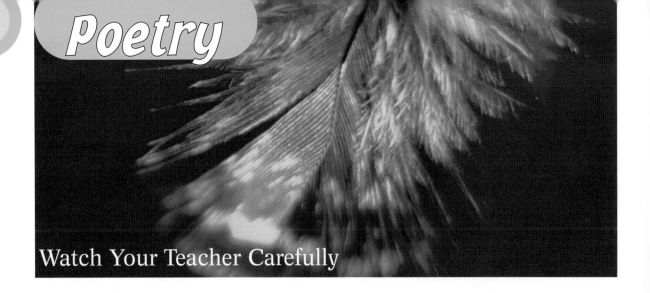

Watch Your Teacher Carefully

It happened in school last week
when everything seemed fine
assembly, break, science, and spelling
three twelves and four times nine.

But then I noticed my teacher
scratching the skin from her cheek
a forked tongue flicked from her lips
her nose hooked into a beak.

Her twenty arms grew longer
they ended in terrible claws
by now she was orange and yellow and green
with crunching great teeth in her jaws.

Her twenty eyes were upon me
as I ran from the room for the Head

got to his office, burst through the door
met a bloodsucking alien instead.

Somehow I got to the staffroom
the doorknob was dripping with slime
inside were seven hideous things
who thought I was dinner time.

I made my escape through a window
just then a roaring sound
knocked me over flat on my face
as the whole school left the ground.

Powerful rockets pushed it
back into darkest space
all I have left are the nightmares
and these feathers that grow on my face.

DAVID HARMER

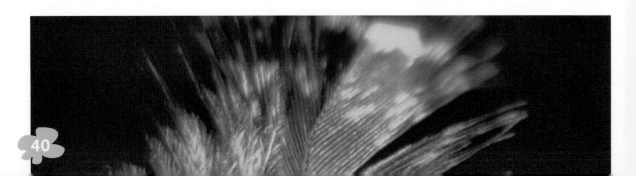

Glossary

alien: a being from another planet
slime: unpleasant slippery stuff
hideous: very ugly

Understanding

1 What is the first thing the narrator notices about his teacher, which makes him think something is wrong?
2 Write down **three** more ways in which his teacher changes.
3 Rewrite the following in your own words: 'inside were seven hideous things who thought I was dinner time'.
4 What does the narrator hear as he escapes through the window? What do you think is making this noise?
5 The last line of the poem tells you that something nasty has happened to the narrator. What has happened and what might happen next?

Extended Writing

1 In the first verse, the word 'fine' rhymes with 'nine'. Find the rhymes in the other six verses. Write a new (last) verse with the same rhyming pattern. Start like this:

Now I have wings like a sparrow
and I live in a nest, in a tree

Add two lines of your own.

2 Imagine the aliens send a short radio message (20 words) back to their own planet. This is how it begins:

MISSION COMPLETE. COMING HOME. SCHOOL CAPTURED.

Complete the message. Try to use the following words:

pupils   teachers   tasty   change   escape

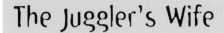

The Juggler's Wife

Last night, in front of thousands of people,

he placed a pencil on his nose

and balanced a chair upright on it

while he spun a dozen plates behind his back.

Then he slowly stood on his head to read a book

at the same time as he transferred the lot

to the big toe of his left foot.

They said it was impossible.

This morning, in our own kitchen,

I ask him to help with the washing-up –

so he gets up, knocks over a chair,

trips over the cat, swears, drops the tray

and smashes the whole blooming lot!

You wouldn't think it was possible.

CICELY HERBERT

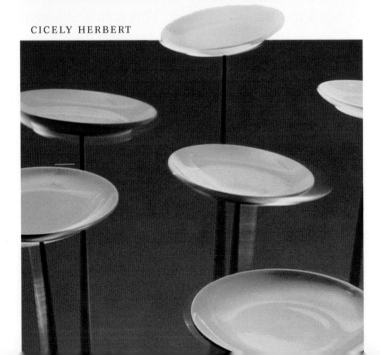

Glossary **transferred:** moved

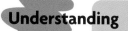**Understanding**

1 What does the juggler balance on his nose?
2 How many plates does he juggle?
3 What does he balance on his big toe?
4 What does he break when he drops the tray?
5 Which phrase tells us that he is famous?
6 Complete the following sentence which sums up how the juggler's wife feels about her husband:

'I think he is a wonderful juggler but ...'

Extended Writing

1 Copy and complete this table.

Job	Something this person does well	Something they do badly
racing driver	drive a fast car	steer a baby buggy
explorer	find hidden treasure	find items in a supermarket
chef	cook fantastic meals	
stuntman/woman		
jet pilot		
famous footballer		

PF 10 **2** Pick one job from the table or choose your own. Write a poem, like 'The Juggler's Wife'. Start the first verse like this:

Last night, in front of ...

The second verse can begin like this:

This morning, in ...

My Christmas; Mum's Christmas

My Christmas	Mum's Christmas
decorations	climbing up to the loft on a wobbly ladder, probably falling.
a Christmas tree	pine needles and tinsel all over the carpet.
lots of food	preparations and loads of dishes to be washed.
crackers	crumpled paper everywhere.
presents	money down the drain.
sweets	indigestion and tooth-ache.
parties	late nights, and driving back through the dark.
snow to play in	getting soaked and frozen whenever outside.

SARAH FORSYTH

Glossary .... **loft:** a room under the roof of a house, an attic
tinsel: strips of glittering material used for decorations
preparations: what has to be done to get ready
indigestion: pain in the stomach caused by eating

Understanding

1 Why might the poet's mum not want to go up into the loft?
2 Which **two** things does she think will create a mess in the house?
3 What does she think will happen if her daughter eats sweets?
4 What, in your own words, is 'money down the drain'?
5 Which part of Christmas does the poet's mother like least? Give a reason for your answer.
6 How old is the poet at the time when she writes this poem? Give reasons for your answer. Use clues from the poem to support your answer.

Extended Writing

1 Write a dialogue between Sarah (the poet) and her mother. Use ideas from the poem and add some of your own. Begin like this:

Sarah: Can we put the Christmas decorations up today, Mum?

Mum: No. I hate going up into the loft. That ladder is dangerous.

Sarah: What about a tree?

PF 11 2 Write a poem like Sarah Forsyth's, entitled 'My Holiday; Grandpa's Holiday'. Use some of these words:

hotel   beach   games   food   night-life

Try to make clear the difference between what you think is a good holiday and what your grandfather thinks.

Good Hot Dogs

Fifty cents apiece
To eat our lunch
We'd run
Straight from school
Instead of home
Two blocks
Then the store
That smelled like steam
You ordered
Because you had the money
Two hot dogs and two pops for here
Everything on the hot dogs
Except pickle lily
Dash those hot dogs
Into buns and splash on
All that good stuff
Yellow mustard and onions
And french fries piled on top all
Rolled up in a piece of wax
Paper for us to hold hot
In our hands
Quarters on the counter
Sit down
Good hot dogs
We'd eat
Fast till there was nothing left
But salt and poppy seeds even
The little burnt tips
Of french fries
We'd eat
You humming
And me swinging my legs

SANDRA CISNEROS

Glossary

cents: American coins (100 cents make one dollar)
pickle lily: child's way of saying piccalilli – a spicy vegetable pickle
quarters: 25-cent coins
poppy seeds: small, black seeds

Understanding

1 How much do the hot dogs cost?
2 How far is the hot dog store from the school?
3 When do the two friends go to the store?
4 What do they order?
5 How old are the two friends? Use clues from the poem to support your answer.

Extended Writing

PF 12 Write a poem, like 'Good Hot Dogs', describing a visit to a fairground. Start like this:

Five pounds each
To go to the fair
We'd run
All the way from home

Use short lines. Use as many of these verbs as you can:

dash   rush   race   spin   roll   fly   twist   turn

Think of an action-filled title.

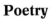

Mama Dot

Born on a sunday
in the kingdom of Ashante

Sold on monday
into slavery

Ran away on tuesday
cause she born free

Lost a foot on wednesday
when they catch she

Worked all thursday
till her hair grey

Dropped on friday
where they burned she

Freed on saturday
in a new century

FRED D'AGUIAR

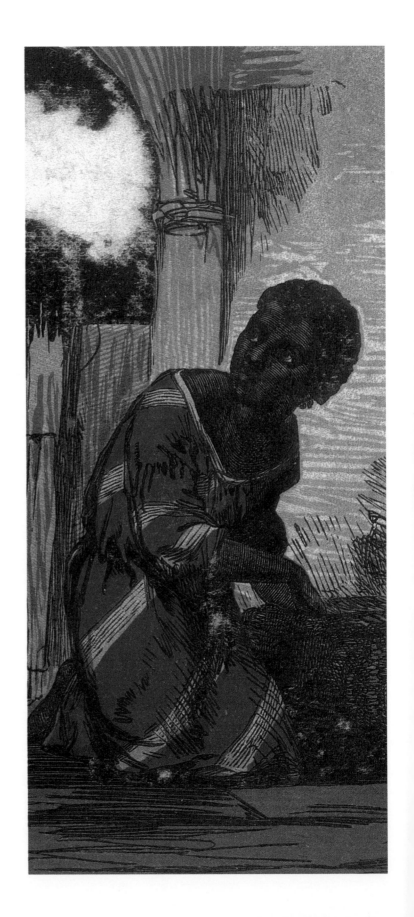

Glossary

Ashante: Part of Africa's west coast (now Ghana)
dropped: died

Understanding

1 On what day was Mama Dot born?
2 What happened to her on Thursday?
3 What, in your own words, does 'Lost a foot' mean?
4 Who are the 'they' who catch Mama Dot? Give a reason for your answer.
5 Does Mama Dot only live for six days? Give a reason for your answer.
6 If she dies ('Dropped') on a Friday, can you think of one way she might be 'freed' on a Saturday?

Extended Writing

1 The poem is a mini-biography (life story) in seven short verses. Use the same structure to write the life story of a fantasy character from a video game or film. You might start like this:

Born on Sunday
in the Kingdom of Fire
Flew on Monday
on wings of flame

Try to think of something dramatic that happens to your character on each day of the week.

2 Expand one of the verses of 'Mama Dot', by adding some details about what might have happened on that day. Write in sentences. For example, the fifth verse could be expanded like this:

On Thursday Mama Dot worked hard all day. She was a slave and had no time to rest. She had very little to eat and drink. She was not an old woman, but her life was so hard her hair went grey.

I Would Run with My Shadow

I would run with my shadow, watch him
    jumping
up at me round a post, peeling himself
    round
railings. Sometimes he'd wriggle
    freely, bumping
over stones without hurting himself;
    sometimes
he was forced to stay bowed, stiffly
    bent, bound
at a wall. With my hands, amazed at his
    mimes,
I'd be a rabbit or wolf. The sunrise
    would stretch
him to a giant and the noon to a blot.
    At sunset
he would hide and be lost. Then a
    switch would fetch
him back. Tables and chairs chopped
    his silhouette
into pieces. A fire was best. He would
    gad
about over the world as if he were mad.

EDMOND LEO WRIGHT

Glossary

bound at a wall: tied to a wall, like a prisoner

mimes: actions without sound

silhouette: a dark shadow seen against a light background

gad about: go about in search of fun

Understanding

1 The poem uses many verbs, such as 'run', 'jumping', 'peeling'. Find **five** more verbs in the poem.

2 What, in your own words, does the poet mean when he says, 'Then a switch would fetch him back'?

3 Describe **two** ways in which the shadow is affected by the sun.

4 What do you think the poet was doing when his shadow stayed 'bowed and stiffly bent'? How did he feel?

5 Why does the poet say 'A fire was best'?

Extended Writing

1 Describe what your shadow does when you:
- run 100-metre race
- do the high jump
- dance at a party.

Use as many verbs in your descriptions as you can.

PF 13 2 Write the first chapter of a story for young children (aged five years and over) entitled 'Me and My Shadow'. Use ideas and words from the poem and your answer to Question 1 (above). Think carefully about your audience. What sort of words will they be able to understand? Will your story be serious or funny?

haircut rap

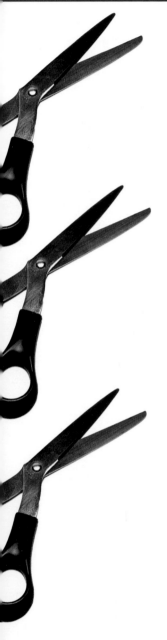

Ah sey, ah want it short,
Short back an' side,
Ah tell him man, ah tell him
When ah teck him aside,
Ah sey, ah want a haircut
Ah can wear with pride,
So lef' it long on top
But short back an' side.

Ah sey try an' put a pattern
In the shorter part,
Yuh could put a skull an' crossbone,
Or an arrow through a heart,
Meck sure ah have enough hair lef'
Fe cover me wart,
Lef' a likkle pon the top,
But the res' – keep it short.

Well, bwoy, him start to cut,
An' me settle down to wait,
Him was cuttin' from seven
Till half-past eight,
Ah was startin' to get worried
Cause ah see it gettin' late,
But then him put the scissors down,
Sey, 'There yuh are, mate.'

Well, ah did see a skull an' a
Criss-cross bone or two,
But was me own skull an bone
That was peepin' through,
Ah look jus' like a monkey
Ah did see once at the zoo,
Him sey, 'What's de matter, Tammy,
Don't yuh like the hair-do?'

Well, ah feel me heart stop beatin'
When me look pon me reflection,
Ah feel like somet'ing frizzle up
Right in me middle section,
Ah look aroun' fe somewhey
Ah could crawl into an' hide
The day ah mek me brother cut
Me hair short back an' side.

VALERIE BLOOM

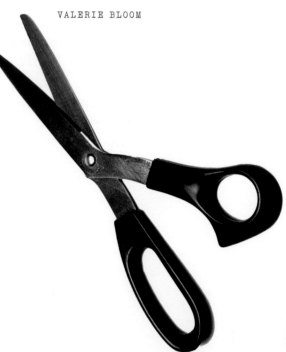

Glossary .... **skull an' crossbone:** the symbol on a pirate flag (skull over crossed bones)

frizzle: shrivel something by burning

Understanding

1 What kind of hair style does Tammy want?
2 Give **one** reason why Tammy does not want her hair cut *very* short.
3 How long does it take Tammy's brother to cut her hair?
4 What, in your own words, does Tammy mean when she says she wants a haircut she can 'wear with pride'?
5 The last verse describes how Tammy feels when she sees herself in the mirror. Summarize the verse, in your own words, in one sentence. Begin like this:

When Tammy sees her hair she feels ...

Extended Writing

1 Make a list of things Tammy could do to try to disguise her new hair cut.

PF 14 2 Write a dialogue between Tammy and her school friend, Ken, when they meet, next day at school. Start like this:

Ken: What happened?

Tammy: What do you mean?

Ken: Your hair. What happened? You been in an accident?

Tammy: That's not funny.

Ken: Who did it?

Tammy: My brother.

Try to include some of your ideas from your answer to Question 1 (above).

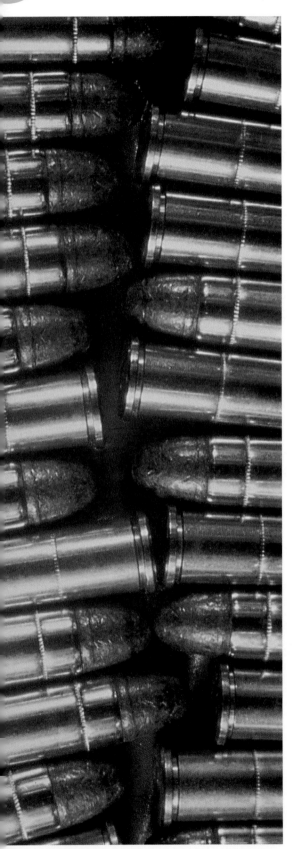

One Question from a Bullet

I want to give up being a bullet

I've been a bullet too long

I want to be an innocent coin

in the hand of a child

and be squeezed through the slot

of a bubblegum machine

I want to give up being a bullet

I've been a bullet too long

I want to be a good luck seed

lying idle in somebody's pocket

or some ordinary little stone

on the way to becoming an earring

or just lying there unknown

among a crowd of other ordinary stones

I want to give up being a bullet

I've been a bullet too long

The question is

Can you give up being a killer?

JOHN AGARD

Glossary

innocent: harmless

idle: not working, doing nothing

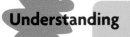

Understanding

1 Which **three** objects would the bullet rather be? Think of **one** thing these three objects have in common.

2 What does the bullet think might happen to the 'ordinary little stone'?

3 The line: 'I've been a bullet too long', has more than one meaning. For instance, it could mean 'I am very old and rusty'. Think of another possible meaning.

4 Why does the poet describe the coin as 'innocent'?

5 The bullet asks a question at the end of the poem. Who is the bullet speaking to?

6 If the bullet could be either a paperclip or a pen knife, which do you think it would choose? Give reasons for your answer.

Extended Writing

1 Write another verse to add to the poem. Use the following beginning:

I want to give up being a bullet.

I've been a bullet too long.

I want to be a ...

Or a ...

And spend my life ...

2 Think of an object and write a short monologue in which this objects speaks. Pick an unusual object (like the bullet); an object that will have some interesting things to say. Try to make the monologue as dramatic as possible. It should have two paragraphs.

Paragraph 1   The object's secret fears.

Paragraph 2   The object's hopes for the future.

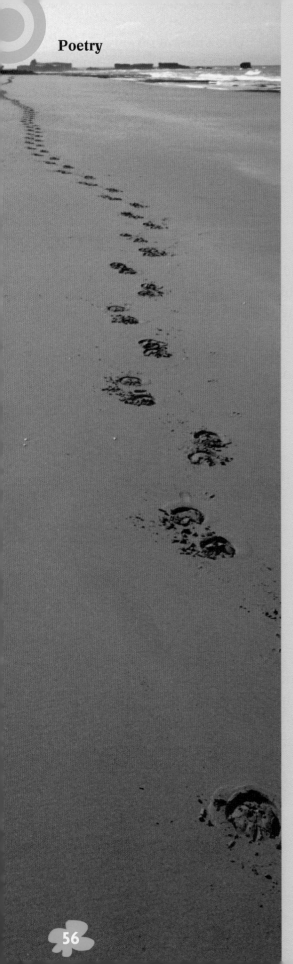

The Sands of Dee

'Oh Mary, go and call the cattle home,
And call the cattle home,
And call the cattle home,
Across the sands of Dee!'
The western wind was wild and dank with foam,
And all alone went she.

The western tide crept up along the sand,
And o'er the sand,
And round and round the sand,
As far as eye could see.
The rolling mist came down and hid the land:
And never home came she.

'O is it weed, or fish, or floating hair –
A tress of golden hair,
A drowned maiden's hair,
Above the nets at sea?'
Was never salmon yet that shone so fair
Among the stakes of Dee.

They rowed her in across the rolling foam,
The cruel crawling foam,
The cruel hungry foam,
To her grave beside the sea;
But still the boatmen hear her call the cattle home,
Across the sands of Dee.

CHARLES KINGSLEY

Glossary

dank: damp and chilly

o'er: over

tress: a lock of hair

stakes: pointed sticks (pushed into the sand to hold a net)

Understanding

1 Why is Mary going across the sands of Dee?

2 Which phrase tells us that she is by herself?

3 When Mary looks around (verse 2) what can she see?

4 How does Mary die? In your own words, what causes her death?

5 What do the last two lines of the poem tell us?

6 In the first verse, the phrase 'call the cattle home' is repeated three times. This helps us to imagine Mary's voice echoing across the sands. Which phrase is repeated in the second verse? Why do you think the poet repeats this phrase?

Extended Writing

1 Use information from the poem to write a short newspaper report about Mary's death. You will need to invent some details, such as her surname, times, dates. Use the following headline and first line.

TRAGIC DROWNING IN RIVER DEE

A young farm-girl was drowned yesterday in the treacherous waters of the River Dee.

PF 15 **2** Write a short epitaph for Mary's gravestone. Include the following information:

Line 1 Her name and age.

Line 2 Where she died.

Line 3 How she died.

You could also add a phrase from the poem.

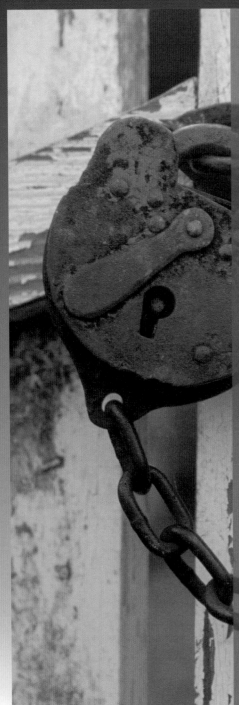

Crying to Get Out

Inside every fat girl
There's a thin girl crying to get out
Sweet and sad and slinky
That nobody ever knows about

Inside every old man
There's a young man crying to get out
Just behind the wrinkles
Is the kid who used to twist and shout

It's the envelope that lies
Only look into their eyes
See the lonely dreamers there
Building castles in the air

Inside every hater
There's a lover dying of the drought
Inside every killer
There's a lover crying to get out
Trying to get out
Dying to get out
All the locked up lovers
Crying to get out

FRAN LANDESMAN

Glossary

slinky: graceful, flowing
twist and shout: dance craze of 1960s
envelope: wrapper, covering
castles in the air: daydreams
drought: a long period of dry weather, a lack of water

Understanding

1 How many times is the word 'every' used in the poem?

2 Complete this sentence:

In the first verse the poet says that all fat girls wish that …

Write a similar sentence for the second verse.

3 Do you agree with what the poet is saying about every fat girl and every old man? Give a reason for your answer.

4 The poet uses a metaphor in the third verse. She compares people to envelopes. What does she mean when she says 'It's the envelope that lies'?

5 The poet could have started her poem like this:

Inside *some* fat girls

There *might be* a thin girl crying to get out

Now rewrite the first verse starting like this:

Inside some fat boys …

6 The poet says that 'nobody ever knows about' what people are hiding inside them. Do you think this is true? Give a reason for your answer.

Extended Writing

1 The poem uses a number of contrasts: fat–thin, old–young, hater–lover. Use a thesaurus to find some more contrasting pairs that the poet might have used.

Use the pairs of words you have found to write sentences like the examples below:

Inside some <u>angry</u> people,

There could be a <u>gentle</u> person crying to get out.

Inside many <u>cruel</u> people,

There may be …

PF 16 2 Write a short pen portrait of a person who has a 'public side' that people see and do not like, but who also has a 'private side' which is much nicer. Write three paragraphs, like this:

Paragraph 1 Describe their public, nasty side.

Paragraph 2 Describe their private, better side.

Paragraph 3 Say why the person hides their better side.

The Rescue

The boy climbed up into the tree.

The tree rocked. So did he.

He was trying to rescue a cat,

A cushion of a cat, from where it sat

In a high crutch of branches, mewing

As though to say to him, 'Nothing doing,'

Whenever he shouted, 'Come on, come down.'

So up he climbed, and the whole town

Lay at his feet, round him the leaves

Fluttered like a lady's sleeves,

And the cat sat, and the wind blew so

That he would have flown had he let go.

At last he was high enough to scoop

That fat white cushion or nincompoop

And tuck her under his arm and turn

To go down –

        But oh! he began to learn

How high he was, how hard it would be,

Having come up with four limbs, to go down with three.

His heart-beats knocked as he tried to think:

He would put the cat in a lower chink –

She appealed to him with a cry of alarm

And put her eighteen claws in his arm.

So he stayed looking down for a minute or so,

To the good ground so far below.

When the minute began he saw it was hard;

When it ended he couldn't move a yard.

So there he was stuck, in the failing light

And the wind rising with the coming of the night.

His father! He shouted for all he was worth.

His father came nearer: 'What on earth – ?'

'I've got the cat up here but I'm stuck.'

'Hold on … ladder …', he heard. O luck!

How lovely behind the branches tossing

The globes of the pedestrian crossing

And the big fluorescent lamps glowed

Mauve-green on the main road.

But his father didn't come back, didn't come;

His little fingers were going numb.

The cat licked them as though to say

'Are you feeling cold? I'm O.K.'

Glossary

crutch: fork in the branches
nincompoop: fool
limbs: arms and legs
chink: a narrow gap or opening
yard: three feet, a distance a little less than one metre
globes: round lights
fluorescent: glowing
numb: unable to feel anything

Understanding

1 Why is the boy climbing the tree?
2 Which lines tell you the wind is strong?
3 The boy climbs up with four limbs. Why must he go down with three?
4 Which lines tell you the cat is terrified she might fall?
5 What can you work out from these lines below about what the boy is feeling?
   'So there he was stuck, in the failing light
   And the wind rising with the coming of the night'.
6 Why is the boy in danger of falling out of the tree?

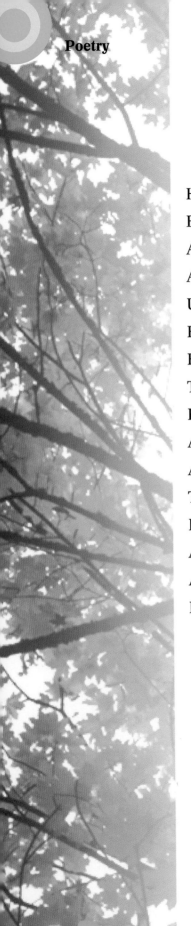

He wanted to cry, he would count ten first,
But just as he was ready to burst
A torch came and his father and mother
And a ladder and the dog and his younger brother.
Up on a big branch stood his father,
His mother came to the top of the ladder,
His brother stood on a lower rung,
The dog sat still and put out its tongue.
From one to the other the cat was handed
And afterwards she was reprimanded.
After that it was easy, though the wind blew:
The parents came down, the boy came too
From the ladder, the lower branch and the upper
And all of them went indoors to supper,
And the tree rocked, and the moon sat
In the high branches like a white cat.

HAL SUMMERS

Glossary   **reprimanded:** told off

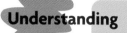

Understanding **7** Who comes to rescue the boy?
8 What part does the dog play in the rescue?
9 Give **one** reason why the poet compares the moon in the high branches with the cat. Try to use some of these words in your answer:

white   high   face   smile   out of reach

Extended Writing

1 Write a sentence about each person involved in the rescue, saying what part they played. You could begin like this:

The boy's brother stood on a lower rung of the ladder, to keep it steady.

The boy's father ...

His mother ...

2 Pick one of the people involved in the rescue. Write a monologue for this person in which they tell a friend or neighbour about the rescue. For example, the mother's monologue might begin like this:

My heart was in my mouth! I nearly had kittens. I looked out of the kitchen window and there was our Scott. Twenty feet up a tree ...

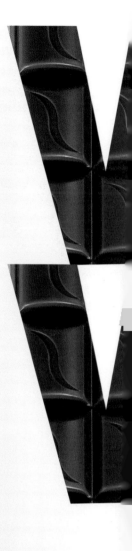

Drama

CHARLIE AND THE CHOCOLATE FACTORY

Charlie Bucket and his family are very poor. Charlie hopes he will find the last Golden Ticket, and win a visit to Willy Wonka's factory, and free chocolate for the rest of his life.

SCENE 3

Bucket home, several days later. Grandparents, Mr and Mrs Bucket, as before.

Mr Bucket	You know, it sure would have been nice if Charlie had won that fifth Golden Ticket.
Mrs Bucket	You mean with that 10p we gave him for his birthday present yesterday?
Mr Bucket	Yes, the one we gave him to buy the one piece of candy he gets every year.
Grandma Georgina	And just think how long it took you two to save that 10p.
Grandpa George	Yes, now that was really a shame.
Grandma Josephine	But think of how Charlie enjoyed the candy. He just loves Willy Wonka chocolate.
Mrs Bucket	He didn't really *act* that disappointed.
Mr Bucket	No, he didn't –
Grandpa Joe	Well, he might not have acted disappointed, but that's because he's a fine boy and wouldn't want any of us to feel sorry for him. Why – what boy wouldn't be disappointed? I sure wish he'd won. I'd do anything for that boy. Why, I'd even –
Charlie	(*Running in excitedly*) Mum! Dad! Grandpa Joe! Grandfolks! You'll never believe it! You'll never believe what happened!

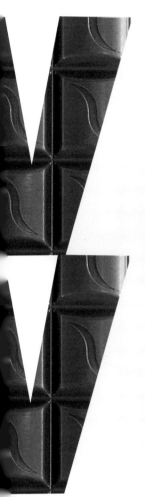

Mrs Bucket	Good gracious, Charlie – what happened?
Charlie	Well … I was walking home … and the wind was so cold … and the snow was blowing so hard … and I couldn't see where I was going … and I was looking down to protect my face … and … and –
Mr Bucket	(*Excitedly*) Go on, Charlie … go on, Charlie … what is it?
Charlie	And there it was … just lying there in the snow … kind of buried … and I looked around … and no one seemed to look as if they had lost anything … and … and … and so I picked it up and wiped it off … and I couldn't believe my eyes –
All (except Charlie)	(*Shouting and screaming*) You found the Golden Ticket! Charlie found the Golden Ticket! Hurray! Hurray! He did it! He did it!

(continued on page 66)

Glossary

candy: sweets, chocolate bars, etc.
disappointed: let down

Understanding

1 How much does Charlie get for his birthday?
2 Who calls Charlie 'a fine boy'?
3 Why, in your own words, is Charlie looking at the ground as he walks home?

Charlie	No … no … I … I found a 50p piece. (*Everybody looks let down and sad*) But, but, but … then I thought it wouldn't hurt if I bought a Wonka Whipple-Scrumptious Fudgemallow Delight since it was … my 50 pence … and I was just *sooo* hungry for one.
All	(*Getting excited again*) Yes … yes … go on … go on.
Charlie	Well … I took off the wrapper slowly … and –
All	(*Shouting and screaming*) YOU FOUND THE GOLDEN TICKET! Charlie found the Golden Ticket! Hurray! Hurray! He did it! He did it!
Charlie	No … no … no … I ate the candy. There wasn't any Golden Ticket. (*Everyone groans and sighs, acting very sad again*) But then … I still had 45 pence left and … well … you know how I love chocolate –
Mrs Bucket	Oh Charlie, you're not sick are you? You didn't spend all of the money on –
Charlie	Well no, as a matter of fact … I bought another Whipple-Scrumptious Fudgemallow Delight … and … and … and I FOUND THE FIFTH GOLDEN TICKET!!!
All	You *what*?
Charlie	I did! I did! I really did! I found the fifth Golden Ticket!!
All	(*Everyone yelling and dancing around*) Hurray! Hurray! Hurray! Yippppppeeeeeeeeeee! It's off to the chocolate factory!!!

RICHARD R. GEORGE
(ADAPTED FROM ROALD
DAHL'S NOVEL)

Understanding   **4** How much money does Charlie find? Where does he find it?
  5 How much does a Fudgemallow Delight cost?
  6 Which lines tell you where the Golden Tickets are hidden?
  7 Describe one way the author makes this scene dramatic and full of suspense.

Extended Writing

In the next scene of the play Grandpa Joe and Charlie set out for Willy Wonka's Chocolate Factory. Write the opening lines of this scene. Think about how Charlie and his grandfather are feeling. Try to get these feelings across in what they say and do. Start like this:

Charlie: *(Pulling Grandpa Joe along at great speed)* Hurry Grandpa. We don't want to be late!

Grandpa Joe: *(Out of breath. Panting)* Slow down ... Charlie ... I need a rest.

Charlie: *(Stopping for a moment)* I wonder what it will be like, Grandpa?

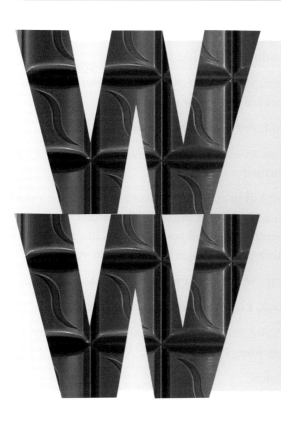

Sitting Pretty

Kate is about to get married. She wants her younger sister, Nicki, a wheelchair user, to be her bridesmaid. But Nicki is not sure if she wants to do this.

Scene 7

The Sitting Room

Kate wheels Nicki back in.

Kate   Mum and Dad will be heartbroken.

Nicki   Yeah, well?

Kate   I'm just saying.

Nicki   They'll get over it.

Kate   But you know what they're like. They've always wanted us to get on, haven't they? You know, like normal sisters.

Nicki   What do you mean 'normal sisters'?

Kate   Well … just … you know.

Nicki   No I don't. I don't know what you mean by 'normal'. Do you mean like normal like sisters who get on really well and never argue with each other? Because I know quite a lot of sisters and they all argue from time to time.

Kate   Yeah, of course they do.

Nicki   So, when you say 'normal' you must mean, what? That one of them isn't disabled.

Kate   I didn't mean it like that.

Nicki   Then you'd better make up your mind what you do mean because that's how it sounded.

Kate   God, you're so angry, aren't you?

Nicki   How would you feel if someone just said that you weren't normal?

Kate   But I didn't say that. Come on, look, I'm on your side. There's no such thing as normal, I know that. It was just a figure of speech. I've heard you say things like that loads of times. I do think you're being a bit over sensitive.

Nicki   Yeah, well maybe I am. Maybe that's how I feel.

Kate   Look, I know you're upset. I'm sorry.

Nicki   It's not your fault. You must hate me. I always take it out on you when I get angry.

Kate   I know.

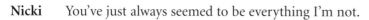

Nicki You've just always seemed to be everything I'm not.

Kate Mum and Dad never treated us like that.

Nicki No, no, they didn't. But I remember one time, when we were … I was about eleven, so you must have been fourteen. You took me over to the park.

Kate Yeah …

Nicki When we got there we 'bumped into' some of your mates. I think you'd planned to meet them and Mum said you couldn't go out unless you took me. There was a boy, Danny.

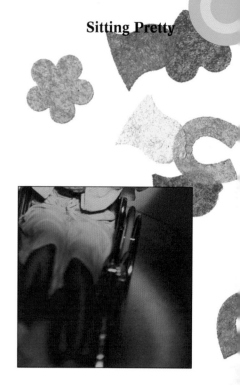

Kate Oh yeah.

Nicki Remember? You left me over by the swings and went and sat on the bench.

Kate I didn't just leave you.

Nicki Then they started, didn't they. Saying things. Calling me names: spastic, cripple, all the usual crap.

Kate And I stuck up for you.

Nicki Yeah, you did. I started crying didn't I? One of them said: 'Look she's crying'. He seemed almost surprised, as if they didn't think I could understand.

Kate I know, it was horrible.

(continued on page 70)

Glossary

heartbroken: very unhappy

figure of speech: a phrase used for dramatic effect, not to be taken literally

over sensitive: easily upset, too sensitive

spastic: used to describe a person with cerebral palsy (no longer used in this way, unless as a term of abuse)

Understanding

1 Why does Kate say 'Mum and Dad will be heartbroken'?

2 Which particular word makes Nicki so angry?

3 Do you think Danny joined in the name calling? Give a reason for your answer.

Nicki   But what you never understood, was that I wasn't crying because of the things that they said. I'd heard them all a thousand times in school, in the street. You get used to that stuff. It probably does less harm than all the pity crap you get on the telly, let's all feel sorry for the poor disabled kid, please send your cheque to this address.

Kate   But it does help a lot of people.

Nicki   No, it gives some people the money they should be getting anyway and turns the rest of us into victims. Disabled people shouldn't be a cause for charity or a way for a bunch of non disabled do gooders to make themselves look good.

Kate   So why were you crying?

Nicki   What's the point, you wouldn't understand.

Kate   Try me.

Nicki   All right. I was crying because, when I got there, I thought … I thought you wanted them to meet me, these were your friends and I thought you wanted me to be there too. Like one of them, these 'normal' people. Then when you just left me by the swings I realized that you didn't want that at all. Not only that, I thought, if that's what it's like, if that's what normal people are like, then I don't want to be like them. But you already were. You stuck up for me because I happened to be your sister and I was upset. But really, you were one of them, and I could never be. I can't blame you for that, but we can never be normal sisters.

Kate   What can I say?

Nicki   Nothing. You didn't choose to have me as a sister. I didn't choose to be like this. But I am. Just don't feel sorry for me because I don't feel sorry for myself. Tell me something, are you happy with the way you are?

Kate   What do you mean?

Nicki   Just that, are you happy with the way you are?

Kate   Well, I wouldn't mind if my bum was a bit smaller, and I wish I'd been a bit cleverer at school, you know, passed a few more exams.

Nicki   So you're not perfect, but you are happy?

Kate   Yes.

Nicki   Good. Me too.

CLIFFORD OLIVER

Glossary   **pity:** feeling sorry

Understanding   **4** Why did Nicki start to cry when she was called names?
5 Nicki calls people who give money to charity 'do gooders'. What does she mean? In your opinion, is she being fair?
6 Why does Nicki say that she and Kate can never be 'normal' sisters?
7 Do you think Nicki is happy? Give a reason for your answer.

Extended Writing

1 If you were acting in this play you would have to say your lines in a certain way to bring out their full meaning. The stage directions in brackets help you to do this. For example:

Nicki   (*Crossly. Turning to look at Kate*) What do you mean 'normal sisters'?

Write stage directions (in brackets) for the following lines:

Kate   Look, I know you are upset. I'm sorry.
Kate   I know, it was horrible.

Now choose some more lines and write directions for those.

PF 17 **2** It is not clear from the extract if Danny joins in the name calling or not. List reasons why Danny might join in. List reasons why he might not. Write a dialogue (with stage directions) between Kate and Danny about the name calling incident.

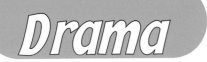

Drama

DREAMS OF ANNE FRANK

Time: 1942, in Amsterdam, Holland, during the Second World War.

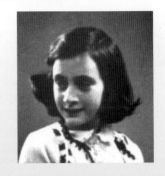

Anne Morning star, evening star, yellow star. Amsterdam. 1942. The German army occupies Holland. They have applied terrible rules that we must obey. Rules for Jews. That applies to me. 'Jews must wear a yellow star. Jews cannot go on trains. Jews must not drive. Jews cannot go shopping, except between three and five. Jews must only patronize Jewish shops.' We cannot go to the cinema, play tennis, go swimming. I cannot even go to the theatre. And now for the most frightening thing of all. They are beginning to round Jews up and take us away. Away from our homes, our beloved Amsterdam. A few days ago I celebrated my thirteenth birthday. My parents gave me this diary. It is my most precious possession. Yesterday I was just an ordinary girl living in Amsterdam. Today I am forced to wear this by our Nazi conquerors. Morning star, evening star, yellow star.

Where are we going to hide? … Will we be alright? … What do I leave behind? … What can I take? … (*Gets her satchel as she hears the answer 'Absolute essentials'*) Essentials. My school satchel. I'm going to cram it full. Hair curlers … Handkerchiefs. School books. Film star photographs. Joan Crawford. Bette Davis. Deanna Durbin. Mickey Rooney. Comb. Letters. Thousands of pencils. Elastic bands. My best book. 'Emil and the Detectives'. Five pens. (*She smells a little bottle*) Nice scent. Oh yes! Mustn't forget my new diary. Have you seen it? … We're going into hiding. (*The others, the family, are all busy packing*) Four days later. It was Thursday the 9th of July. I shall never forget that morning. It was raining. Imagine leaving your house, maybe forever … Goodbye, house … We'll always remember you … Thank you for everything. My brain is at a fairground, on a roller-coaster. Up and down. Happy. Sad. Afraid. Excited …

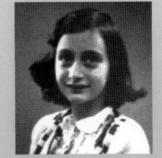

BERNARD KOPS

Glossary

occupies: takes over using force, invades
patronize: use, spend money at
essentials: things we cannot do without

Understanding

1 In what year does the German army take over Anne's country?

2 Write down **two** of the 'Rules for Jews' – one which affects **where** Anne can go and one which affects **when** she can go.

3 How old is Anne? Use a quotation to support your answer.

4 Why is she leaving her home?

5 Where is she going?

6 Why, in your own words, does she feel as if her 'brain is at a fairground, on a roller-coaster'?

Extended Writing

1 Read through the extract again. Write down any words and phrases that give you a clue about Anne's feelings. Begin like this:

'terrible rules that we must obey'

'the most frightening thing of all'

'Will we be alright?'

PF 18 **2** Anne's diary is her 'most precious possession'. In it she writes down all her secret hopes and fears. Write a diary entry for the day she leaves her home and goes into hiding. Try to show how she was feeling. Use words and phrases from Question 1 (above). Begin like this:

Amsterdam

Thursday 9th July 1942

Today I left the house that has been my home ever since I can remember. Now everything has changed. I am so sad and afraid. Today was a wet, grey day. As if the clouds were weeping too …

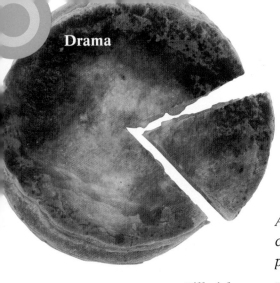

SUPERMARKET CHECKOUT

*An impatient woman **customer** is having her groceries checked out by a slow **girl** on the till. She looks at a packet of bacon.*

Till girl   It's got no price on. Did you notice how much they were?

Customer   No, I didn't.

Till girl   *She looks round and holds up the bacon.*

Won't be long.

Customer   Good.

Long pause.

Till girl   We're a bit short-handed today. Us that works here gets the old food cheap, and if it's something like a pork pie, you can actually die, apparently. So the girl that checks the prices, she's probably, you know, passed on.

Customer   Honestly, I thought you girls on the tills knew all the prices.

Till girl   I've only come on the till today. I was in meat packing before, then an overall came free so I come here.

Customer   But surely you wear an overall when you're packing meat?

Till girl   No, you must bring something from home. I had our dog's blanket.

Customer   You can't have a dog in a place where food is prepared.

Till girl   I didn't. It's dead. It were called Whiskey. It ate one of the pork pies from here.

Customer   But you do wear gloves don't you, when you're wrapping meat?

Till girl   I did, woolly ones. I get a lot of colds, I like to have something to wipe my nose on. I liked it in the meat-packing department, it were dead near the toilet.

Customer	Well it sounds disgusting. Who's in charge of that department?
Till girl	Mr Waterhouse. He's not here. He goes to some sort of special clinic on Thursdays. I'll do your veg, anyway.
	She coughs and splutters all over it.
Till girl	Sorry, I've caught this cold off Susan on smoked meats. They're not smoked when they come, but she's on sixty a day.
Customer	It's all over the cauliflower.
Till girl	Sorry.
	She wipes it on her overall.
Till girl	Corned beef, ninety-eight. It's funny how much tins can actually blow out without bursting, isn't it?
Customer	You can't sell a blown tin.
Till girl	We can, they're dead popular.

(continued on page 76)

Glossary

short-handed: very busy, because other assistants are away
passed on: died

Understanding

1 Why is the till girl holding up a packet of bacon?
2 How long has the till girl been working on the check-out?
3 Why does she like to wear gloves when she is packing meat?
4 Write down **three** things you learn from the sketch about Susan.
5 How much is the corned beef?

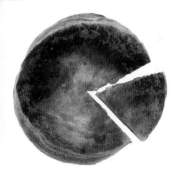

Customer	Oh look, how much longer is this going to take?
Till girl	Do you want me to ask the supervisor?
Customer	Yes, thank you.
	The till girl speaks into intercom.
Till girl	Hello?
Intercom	Hello?
Till girl	Hello, Mrs Brinsley, it's Gemma here.
Intercom	Hello Gemma, nice to talk to you.
Till girl	Nice to talk to you, Mrs Brinsley. How's your boils?
Intercom	Worse.
Till girl	So putting you on the cheese counter hasn't helped? Well, what I'm calling about, I've a lady here, and she's brought me a packet of bacon with no price.
Intercom	Is it streaky?
Till girl	Well it is a bit but it'll probably wash off.
	She wipes it with a filthy dishcloth.
Till girl	The sell-by-date is 5 August 1984. No, hang on.
	She scrapes something off.
Till girl	1964.
Intercom	Three and nine.
Till girl	Three and nine, thank you.
Customer	You mean the bacon is twenty years old?
Till girl	I don't know. I was away when we did addings.
	She finishes checking the rest of the stuff.
Customer	This place is a disgrace – filthy, unhygienic, the food's not safe to eat, the staff are all positively diseased.
Till girl	That's two pounds seventy-one pence, please.
Customer	On the other hand, it's very cheap and easy to park. Bye.

VICTORIA WOOD

Glossary

supervisor: person in charge
unhygienic: dirty, full of germs

Understanding

6 What is the till girl's name?
7 What is the sell-by-date on the bacon? How old is the bacon?
8 Give **two** reasons why the customer thinks the supermarket is a disgrace.
9 What does the last line of the sketch tell you about the customer?

Extended Writing

1 Read the sketch again. Make a list of anything that goes on in the supermarket which might harm the health of customers and staff. Begin like this:

Staff can buy old (out-of-date) food cheap.
Staff are not given the correct overalls.'

2 You are the next customer at the same check-out. You are so disgusted by what you hear you demand to see the supervisor, Mrs Brinsley. Write a dialogue between you and the supervisor. Include the following words:

angry   complain   sell-by-date   rotting   smelly
germs   disease   Black Death   police   sorry
goodbye

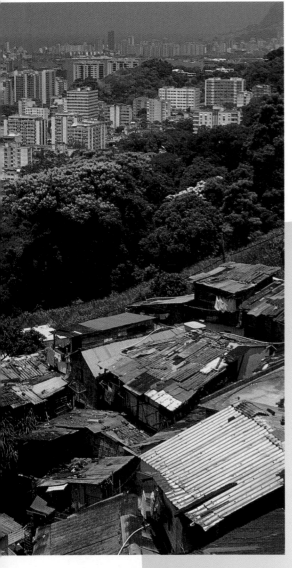

Mariza's Story

This play is set in the present day, in a large modern city, surrounded by shanty towns. Mariza, her mother and sister go into the city centre each day, to try to make a little money.

Act 1
Scene 1

*Mariza, eight years old, her **Mum**, in her thirties, and her sister **Tania**, twelve, walking at night along a road. Traffic goes past. They have been walking for hours. **Mum** and **Tania** carry sacks on their heads. **Mariza** falls behind.*

She is wearing an old coat and has a battered doll in her hand.

Very tired, they stop and put down their loads.

They are dusty, dressed in old clothes and have bare feet.

*Tania sits on the sack, soon imitated by **Mariza** who sits on her mum's sack.*

Tania	Mum, look! The bus.
Mum	We don't have money for tickets.
	Mariza goes towards the bus.
Mum	Mariza!
Tania	Get back here!
	They carry on walking. Again, they stop even more tired than before.
Mum	It's a long way to go home.
Tania	Another four miles.
Mariza	Another four miles.

Tania	You shut up.
Mum	Come on, let's try.
Tania	Mum, wait.

Tania tries hailing cars, without any luck.

	With so many cars going by … with so many lorries and buses … why can't we take one?
Mum	I told you, Tania, we haven't got the money for the tickets.
Tania	Aren't people kind?
Mum	Not to those like us.
Tania	We are people just like everyone else, aren't we?
Mum	I know, Tania. But we are not like them.
Tania	Why aren't we like people with cars, Mum?
Mum	We're street people. They're car people. Come on. Let's try to cover another stretch. I'm worried about our home.

Glossary

imitated: copied

hailing cars: calling out to passing cars, trying to get them to stop

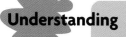

Understanding

1 What is Tania carrying? What is her sister carrying?
2 How far are they from their home?
3 What do you think the mother means when she says: 'We're street people. They're car people'?

*They walk on again, **Mariza** losing ground. Her **Mum** sees her and stops.*

Tania	Don't stop now.
Mum	Tania. Mariza's too small to walk for so long.
Tania	She's too heavy to be carried.

Mum ties a rope around Mariza's waist.

Mum	I don't want to lose you. It's a dark night.

(continued on page 80)

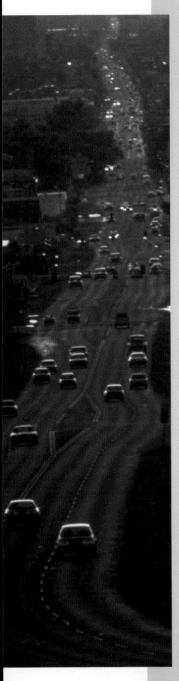

Tania tries flagging down more cars. Again without any luck.

Mum   Come on, let's walk on.

Tania   But it's too far!

Mum   We have done this road yesterday. And the day before, and before … To town and back.

Tania   How come tonight we can't do it?

Mariza starts crying.

Mum   She's hungry.

Tania   We haven't eaten anything today, have we?

Mum   Yes, it's harder tonight. We have eaten less and less each day.

Tania   Yes, but today nothing at all.

Tania puts her load down.

Tania   I can't do it Mum. I'd rather die here.

Mum   Look, Tania, rest a bit here with your little sister. I'll walk on, on my own. It's important I get home. We left it this morning with nobody looking after it. There's so many thieves about. You can't leave your house on its own any longer. Our house is all we have.

Tania   Go ahead then.

Mum hands the end of the rope to Tania.

Mum   Make your way a little at a time. Watch yourselves from strangers.

Tania   Yes, Mum.

Mum walks away. Mariza cries. Tania calms her. Then Tania and Mariza resume walking. Mariza stops.

Tania   Come on.

Mariza   It's dark.

Tania   It's night, that's why.

Mariza   It's getting darker, Tania.

Tania   It's your eyes, Mariza. Please, don't fall asleep.

Mariza collapses. Tania speaks angrily, to herself.

Tania   Oh, how can we walk like this! We must get home. Maybe if they see a child, one of the cars will stop.

Tania holds Mariza in front of her as she tries to stop the passing traffic. Then, the braking noise of a car is heard.

Tania   Oh! It's stopped. We're lucky, Mariza!

The driver comes up to them and looks them up and down.

MICHELE CELESTE

Glossary

losing ground: falling behind
flagging down: stopping a car by waving at it
resume: restart, carry on
collapses: falls down

Understanding

4 What does Mum do to keep Mariza safe?
5 Why do they feel weak and tired?
6 Why does Mum leave the two girls and go on by herself?

Extended Writing

1 Read both scenes again. Write down any clues that tell you that life for Mum and her girls is hard and sometimes dangerous. Begin like this:

They have to walk along a busy road in the dark.
They have to carry heavy sacks.

2 Imagine you are a street kid. You are one of thousands of homeless youngsters living on the streets in the same city where Mariza and Tania live. Describe how you became a street kid. Did you run away? How do you find food? Where do you sleep? Use your list for Question 1 to help you. Begin like this:

My name is … . I am fourteen years old. I have been a street kid for … years. I had to leave my home because …

Stocking-fillers

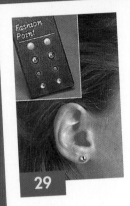

29 Stick-on Earrings

You don't need pierced ears to wear these tiny studs – they look like the real thing, but simply stick on. Can be used over and over again. 4 elegant pairs with crystal, pearl, silver and gold effect finishes. Perfect for nose studs too! Not a toy.
£1.95 set

304 Key Finder Torch

Never lose your keys again. Just whistle, and Key Finder will beep and flash from anywhere in the room, helping you to find your keys immediately. Also a handy light for locating keyholes in the dark. Battery supplied.
£5.95 each

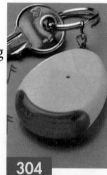

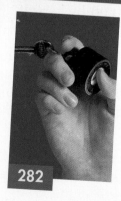

282 Personal Alarm

Arguably every teenager should carry one of these. Our new model is an extra tiny size but an even louder 130 decibels, activated simply by pressing through the base of the alarm. Spare energy cell included.
3.7cm diam.
£5.95 each

Glossary

effect: coloured to look like

decibels: a measurement of how loud a sound is (as height is measured in centimetres)

activated: turned on

locating: finding

Understanding

1 How many pairs of stick-on earrings do you get in a set? How many different colours?

2 Which phrase tells you they can be used more than once?

3 Why do you think the advert includes the phrase 'Not a toy'?

4 How do you set off the personal alarm?

5 State **two** ways in which the new alarm model is different from the old model.

6 Say, in your own words, how the Key Finder Torch works.

Extended Writing

1 All three adverts contain facts about each product. For example, the torch has a battery supplied with it. All the adverts also contain opinions about the products. For example, the advert for the Key Finder Torch suggests that if you buy one of these torches you will never lose your keys again. Copy and complete the table below.

Product	Facts	Opinions
Stick-on Earrings	can be used as nose studs	
Personal Alarm		
Key Finder Torch		

PF 19 2 Pick one of the products below and write a short advert (50 words maximum) for it. Include facts about the product, for example, its price, size, colour, age range, etc. Also include some opinions, for example, 'Every teenager must have one ...'

• Musical socks (socks which play a tune when you walk about in them)

• Colour change yo-yo (yo-yo with flashing lights inside it)

• Glow in the dark glasses.

The Worst Row I Ever Had

'When I was seven my oldest brother took my favourite doll and buried it in a field near our house. When they found out, my parents dragged him around for hours trying to find the spot where he'd put it. But they couldn't. I was so angry I wouldn't speak to him or even look at his face, and even though my mum and dad pleaded with me and eventually even shouted at me to make up with him, I wouldn't. Then after four months I finally just got fed up with it and one night when we were having tea I spoke to him. My dad was so surprised he nearly choked on a piece of pork chop!'

Catherine, 12

'When I was nine I had a row with my dad because I wanted to take this computer toy I'd been given to school to show off to everyone and he wouldn't let me in case it got broken or stolen. It was stupid really, but I got so worked up about it I called him lots of names. I said he was fat and ugly and I wished he wasn't my dad. Then, I went to his and Mum's room and tore up his favourite picture of him that I'd painted in nursery school. When I got home from school at the end of that day my auntie was waiting there to tell me that Dad had been in a car accident and was in hospital. Luckily he wasn't badly hurt and soon got better, but since then if ever I argue with someone, I always try to make-up with them straight away, because you never know otherwise if it might be too late.'

Rebecca, 14

Glossary

eventually: in the end
worked up: very upset

Understanding

1 Who did Catherine have her row with?
2 When did the row happen – how many years ago?
3 How did she behave towards her brother?
4 Which phrase tells you that Catherine's parents begged her to end the row?
5 Give **one** reason why Catherine's dad was so surprised when the row ended.
6 What did Rebecca want to take to school? Why did this cause a row?
7 Who was waiting for Rebecca when she got home from school?
8 How did Rebecca feel when she got the bad news?

Extended Writing

1 Describe the row over the doll through Catherine's brother's eyes. Begin like this:

When I was twelve I took my little sister Catherine's favourite doll. I buried it in a field near our house. When they found out, my parents ...

2 Write about a row you have had. Describe what it was about, how it was settled and how you feel about it now.

Human Interest Stories

Boy, 9, rides 150 miles under lorry

BY TOM LEONARD

A NINE-year-old boy who has run away 30 times in the past year was found almost 150 miles from his home yesterday after wedging himself under a lorry.

Aaron Bowers, who has hitched a ride in the same way three times in a week, was reported missing from his home in Stoke-on-Trent, Staffs, on Monday. The next day he was discovered in a garden in the village of Spennithorne, near Leyburn, North Yorks.

His father, Colin Bowers, 43 – a lorry driver – said the family were at their wits' end. 'Each time he goes a bit further and each time we think we won't see him again.'

A police spokesman said: 'After a clean-up, the lad appeared unscathed. He told us he had travelled from Stoke hidden above the back axle of a heavy lorry.'

The boy said at the weekend that he 'just liked the excitement'.

from the *Daily Telegraph*

SON SAVES SICK FATHER

A BOY of 10 grabbed the wheel of his dad's car and brought it to a stop after he had a diabetic attack.

Joshua Hardcastle steered the Citroen safely on to a grass verge then flagged down help.

He said: 'I was very scared but I knew I had to get help.

'I know lots about cars, so I had no problem moving it off the road.'

He noticed father Peter was unwell when he started slurring his speech.

Peter, 44, said: 'I had a can of cola in my pocket which I usually keep for emergencies but because we were caught in traffic I was unable to drink it.'

Joshua took control, stopped the car and put on the handbrake.

He then stopped a passing motorist who took them to a farmhouse nearby where Peter, of Ossett, West Yorks, had his drink.

Both were given the all clear after hospital check-ups.

from the *Daily Mirror*

Glossary

unscathed: without being injured

axle: metal rod or bar on which a wheel turns

diabetic attack: fainting fit brought on by a lack of sugar

Citroen: make of car

flagged down: stopped a car by waving at it

slurring: speaking unclearly, jumbling words

Understanding

1 How old is Aaron?

2 Write down **three** more facts about Aaron.

3 Why, in your own words, are Aaron's family at their 'wits' end'?

4 Give your opinion of what Aaron did. Complete this sentence:

I think what Aaron did was … because …

5 How old is Joshua?

6 Which phrase tells you how he felt when his father became unwell?

7 What **two** things did Joshua do as soon as he saw his father was ill?

8 In your own words, what caused the incident?

Extended Writing

1 Write a sentence about both boys. Describe how they felt when they saw the newspaper reports. Begin like this:

I think Aaron might have been …

PF 20 **2** Write a short newspaper report about an incident involving a young person. Try to copy the style of the reports opposite.

Paragraph 1 Tell the reader briefly what has happened.

Paragraph 2 Give details of the young person's family, school, home town, etc.

Paragraph 3 Include comments by the youngster and/or his or her family about the incident.

Pick one of these headlines or invent one of your own.

GIRL, 12, RESCUES CAT FROM FLOODED RIVER

BOY IN MIRACLE LIGHTNING ESCAPE

A day in the life of RSPCA veterinary surgeon Tessa Bailey – of Animal Hospital ...

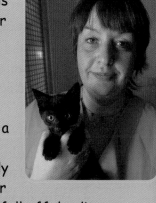

8 am As I arrive the waiting room is already busy. Patients checking in for operations and some 'early birds' for clinic. Summer is a busy time at the hospital.

8.30 am During ward rounds I check on any new arrivals. Bouncer – a big, shaggy cross-bred dog – is seriously injured. His owners foolishly left him alone on the balcony of their fourth-floor home and poor Bouncer fell off, landing on the concrete car park below. He has broken both front legs and his jaw, and is bleeding inside, which could be fatal. He is attached to a special drip to replace lost blood and will be X-rayed later when he improves.

10 am Vets Julie and Liz are busy with flea and cat flu problems. It is frustrating to see animals suffer when it could have easily been avoided with regular treatment.

11.30 am Great news! Bouncer's X-rays show the bleeding has stopped. I bandage strips of wood – called splints – to his legs, which keep his broken bones straight and the nurses will keep him comfortable day and night with painkillers. Tomorrow I will fix metal plates in his legs and jaw to mend the bones. He is lucky to be alive.

3 pm A Staffordshire bull terrier is rushed in. He is gasping for breath and his tongue is blue. I immediately give him oxygen and take his temperature – it is extremely high. This dog has heat stroke and unless we quickly cool him down, he will die. I immediately cover him with cold water and ice, inject fluids to stop him getting dehydrated, and give him medication to keep his blood circulating. We save him, but only just.

Heat stroke is a common problem with animals in the summer, so please make sure your pets have plenty of shade and water and never leave an animal in a car.

5 pm Time to go home and check my own rabbits, Flopsy and Bunnita, and think about what lies ahead tomorrow.

FROM THE RSPCA'S **ANIMAL ACTION** MAGAZINE

Glossary

early birds: people who arrive early
shaggy: long-haired
cross-bred: mongrel
fatal: cause death
dehydrated: lacking in water
medication: medicines
circulating: flowing around the body

Understanding

1 At what time does Tessa start work?
2 Who are Julie and Liz?
3 How is Bouncer injured?
4 Which word tells you that Bouncer might die?
5 Which phrases tell you that the Staffordshire bull terrier is very close to dying?
6 Tessa works hard all day. At what time do you think she is busiest? Give a reason for your answer.

Extended Writing

1 Copy and complete the table below.

Animal	Problem	Cause
dog (Bouncer)		owners' foolishness
cats	flu and fleas	
dog (bull terrier)		

2 Write down what Tessa says when she returns Bouncer to his owners. Write three paragraphs like this:
Paragraph 1 Tessa tells the owners about Bouncer's injuries.
Paragraph 2 She describes how the injuries were treated.
Paragraph 3 Tessa tells the owners why the dog was hurt, and what they must do in future to avoid a similar accident.

*your*shout!

In our January issue, we told you about a reader's dilemma. Here's what you said she should do …

this month's problem

She keeps asking me for money

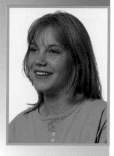

I've been best mates with Kelly since I was four, but recently our relationship's been under a lot of strain.

Kelly keeps asking me to lend her money and although it's never more than a couple of quid at a time, she never pays me back. I don't like to ask in case I sound stingy, but I'm beginning to resent Kelly for taking liberties with me. What should I do?

Liza, 15

Be tough!

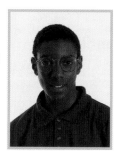

This girl's taking you for granted and it's about time you gave her a wake-up call! When you borrow money from someone, you should always return it, no matter how small the amount.

If she's taking advantage of you, it's a sign she doesn't respect your friendship. Talk to her calmly, but be firm.

Ken, 18

Act now

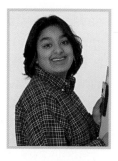

Don't let her take advantage of you! I understand it's difficult to make a point about it, because you don't want to upset Kelly. But if you continue acting like nothing's wrong, the problem will get worse. Act now, before it's too late!

Yiljan, 19

Don't give in

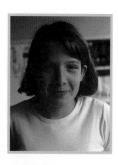

Sooner or later, you're going to have to tell it to Kelly like it is. If you keep on lending her money without ever getting it back, the situation is just going to get worse and worse. Don't worry about confronting her about it. If she's a truly good friend, she'll understand your point of view. Just make sure you remember one thing – it's *your* money, not hers!

Angela, 13

FROM **SUGAR** MAGAZINE

Glossary

stingy: mean
taking liberties: going too far, overstepping the mark
take advantage of: take for granted, use
a wake-up call: a shock
confronting: facing up to

Understanding

1 How old is Liza? For how long has she been friends with Kelly?
2 Why is Liza upset with Kelly?
3 Why does Yiljan tell Liza to act now before it is too late?
4 Which phrase do both Yiljan and Ken use? What does it mean?
5 Do you agree with what Ken says about borrowing money? Give a reason for your answer.
6 Re-read what Liza says about Kelly. Angela says Liza should confront Kelly. What does she mean by this? Do you think Liza will take Angela's advice? Give a reason for your answer.

Extended Writing

1 Rewrite Liza's problem as a third person narrative. Begin like this:

THIS MONTH'S PROBLEM

Kelly keeps asking Liza for money. Liza has been mates with Kelly since she was four, but recently their relationship's been under a lot of strain.

Kelly keeps asking her …

2 Re-read what Yiljan, Ken, and Angela say to Liza. Pick out any phrases which tell Liza to be strong and do something about the problem. Begin like this:

'Act now, before it's too late!'

Write down what you would say to Liza about her problem. Use some of the phrases from your list.

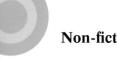

Cool Spoons

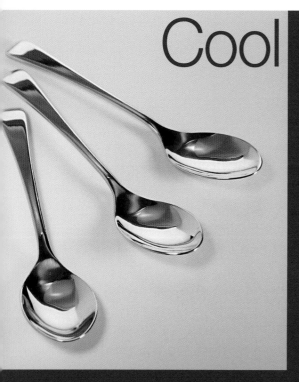

THE EFFECT

The magician can tell which of three spoons has been chosen by a member of the audience, simply by touching them.

YOU NEED

- Three metal teaspoons
  (it's best if you leave them in the fridge for a few minutes before the trick)

- A blindfold

TO PERFORM

Lay the spoons out in a row and put on the blindfold. Ask someone to pick one up. Tell them you are going to tell which spoon they've chosen by reading their mind. Ask them to press it against their forehead with the palm of their hand for 20 seconds or so, to help transmit the mental waves, then put it down.

Pick up each spoon in turn, secretly feeling the temperature, and saying, 'Now was it this one … or this one … or this one? I think it was this one!'

Hold up the warmest spoon. They'll be amazed.

WHAT HAPPENED

While they hold the spoon in their hand their body heat is conducted into the metal, so the spoon gets warmer.

FROM **CONJURING IN THE KITCHEN** BY RICHARD ROBINSON

Glossary

transmit: send

mental waves: messages from the mind or brain

conducted: passed

Understanding

1 What do you need to do this trick?

2 What does the other person do once the magician is blindfolded?

3 Why does the other person need to press the spoon against their forehead for 20 seconds?

4 Write down **one** thing that could make the trick go wrong.

5 Say, in your own words, how the trick works. Write a sentence starting like this:

The magician can tell which spoon the other person picked because ...

Extended Writing

Write a monologue for a magician performing the Cool Spoons trick. Begin like this:

Ladies and gentlemen, boys and girls, I am Presto the Magician. I am going to do a truly amazing trick. All I need are three spoons and this blindfold. First, I place the spoons on the table, like this. Next I put on my extra thick blindfold. Now ...

Horror Story Reviews

VAMPIRE STORIES TO TELL IN THE DARK

ANTHONY MASTERS

Short stories about vampires told by a group of teenagers spending an evening in a crypt.

'Exciting and very scary.'
Michelle Gray

CAMP FEAR

CAROL ELLIS

Eight teenagers acting as counsellors at Summer Camp are being terrorized by fears of an accident that happened seven years ago. They are worried that history is going to repeat itself, and their worst nightmares will materialize.

'The book made me edgy and uncomfortable – it was quite scary, even bone-chilling in parts.'
Donna Lane

LOCH

PAUL ZINDEL

Rumours of a great black beast in the waters of a remote lake in Vermont have led a team of 'researchers' to hunt for it. The team leader is determined to destroy the creature but Loch and his sister are equally determined that this shouldn't happen.

'A really good horror story – tense, exhilarating, full of suspense and adventure – it has everything.'
Daniel Shurville

THE FEAR MAN

ANN HALAM

14-year-old Andrei is constantly moving house with his mother to avoid meeting his estranged father. One day he is drawn to a house, where he seems to disturb someone or something. From then on he starts seeing the Fear Man.

'This is really scary because you are not sure who or what the Fear Man is. It sent chills down my spine and I just had to keep reading. Great cover too.'
Polly Robinson

FRANKENSTEIN

MARY SHELLEY

The classic tale of the man-made monster come to life and the trail of destruction, human and material, that follows in its wake.

'Very creepy and tense. I don't normally like horror stories, but I was totally engrossed, especially when the monster threatens his creator. Reading this has made me want to try other horror stories.'
Clare Darling

Glossary

crypt: a room under a church often used as a burial chamber
counsellors: people who give advice or help
terrorized: frightened
materialize: become real
edgy: tense
bone-chilling: very frightening
remote: far away, distant
exhilarating: very exciting
estranged: kept apart, having once been friendly or loving
engrossed: involved

Understanding

1 Which story is about a creature that lives in a lake?
2 Who reviews a story about a summer camp?
3 In *Camp Fear* the teenagers are anxious that 'history is going to repeat itself'. What, in your own words, does this mean?
4 Explain why Daniel liked *Loch*.
5 Which story is described as a classic tale? What does the word 'classic' mean?
6 What do you think happens to the creature in *Loch*?

Extended Writing

1 Make a list of all of the words and phrases used in the reviews to describe horror stories. Begin like this:

exciting

scary

PF 21 2 Write a short review of a book or film which you think is scary. Start by stating the title of the film or book. Then give a brief plot summary. Then write your review, saying what you thought of it.

True Stories of
Tots and Toddlers

Extract A

One Sunday when my daughter Monique was coming up to four, we drove down to Littlehampton.

After forty-five miles of her repeatedly asking 'Are we there yet?', I pointed to a huge blue sign board and read out loud, 'Welcome to Littlehampton.'

There was a short pause.

'Did that sign really say that, Daddy?'

'Yes,' I said. 'Why?'

'How did they know we were coming?' she replied, mystified.

CLIVE KAVANAGH

Extract B

Roanne and Steven are my step-grandchildren. They were visiting, and the three of us were sitting in the garden. The conversation went like this:

Roanne: 'Barbara, why have you got a dish of dog food in the garden under the trees?'

Me: 'It's there for my hedgehog. He likes dog food.'

Roanne: 'If we are very quiet, might we see him?'

Me: 'I don't think so, dear. He sleeps in the day and only wakes up at night' ... I thought they might know the word "nocturnal" so I added, 'Do you know what we call someone who does that?'

Roanne: 'No, I don't.'

Steven: 'I do, Barbara. They are called burglars.'

BARBARA GODFREY

Extract C

Our son, Ian, who could swim, was playing in the pool with a polystyrene float. At one point, he slipped from this into the water, which was very cold.

An asthmatic, he lost his breath, and being then unable to shout, he was going under for the third time when he was spotted by the lifeguard and a friend who both dived into the pool to his rescue.

The lifeguard took Ian to the shower-room to get him warmed up.

Ian, no worse for his experience, was chatting away with him.

The lifeguard explained that he would normally provide people like Ian with a drink, but went on to say that because it was so early in the season he had no stock of drinks, so would Ian like a glass of water instead.

'Don't you think I've had enough water already?' Ian replied.

WIN AND NEIL MORLEY

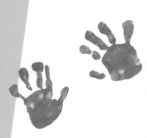

From **The Terrible Twos: True Stories of Tots and Toddlers** compiled by Sarah Kennedy

Glossary

repeatedly asking: asking over and over again

mystified: puzzled, confused

nocturnal: active at night, sleeping during the day

an asthmatic: someone with asthma, a disease that makes breathing difficult

Understanding

1 How old was Monique?
2 Who was she travelling with? Where were they going?
3 Why does Barbara put a bowl of dog food in her garden?
4 When Barbara asked the question, 'Do you know what we call someone who does that?' what answer did she expect? Why do you think Steven gave the answer he did?
5 How is Barbara related to Roanne and Steven?
6 Where was Ian when the accident happened?
7 Why did the lifeguard take him to the shower-room?

Extended Writing

1 Carry on the dialogue between Barbara and Steven (Extract B). Begin like this:

Barbara: (Laughing) No! Not burglars! A creature that sleeps in the day and wakes up at night is nocturnal.

Steven: Well, burglars go out at night. I saw it on 'Crimewatch'.

Barbara: That's different.

Steven: Why is it different?

Barbara: Because …

2 Rewrite Extract C as a first person narrative, through the eyes of the lifeguard. Begin like this:

I was on duty at the pool last week when a little lad called Ian Morley got into difficulties. He was playing on a float when he slipped into the water. The water was very cold …

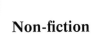

Coping with Girls: Gifts

The trick is to suit the gift to the situation. Here are some examples:

At the pictures

Good gift: Sweets or chocolates. But nothing crackly or sticky There's nothing worse than not being able to hear the film for the rustle of paper, or hold her hand without getting covered in dribbly chocolate. And if you buychocolates, make sure she isn't on a diet.

Bad gift: A bunch of flowers. Where is she going to stick them all through the film?

At her house

If you're invited round to her house … then the gift is very important.

Good gift: A bunch of flowers, but check first she doesn't suffer from hay fever! You don't want her sneezing and dribbling all over your best clobber, do you? But flowers are a great idea, as they'll impress her parents. Also, her whole family can have a sniff, which saves buying anything separate for them.

Bad gift: A magazine on wrestling. It could give her parents quite the wrong (or right!) idea about what the pair of you are going to get up to if you're left alone for five minutes!

At a restaurant

Good gift: A single rose. But leave the price tag on. This is so the waiter won't think you've pinched it out of the vase on the table!

Bad gift: Anything edible. This could spoil her appetite. Although if she's a big eater, then a medium sliced loaf could come in very handy and save you a fortune …

At the disco

Good gift: Perfume. A little dab after a bit of dancing could prove very welcome. For you, as well as the girl! But when I say perfume, I do mean perfume. We are not talking underarm deodorant here!

Bad gift: A bag of marbles … She might drop them and cause a major pile-up.

FROM **THE A TO Z OF COPING WITH GIRLS/BOYS** BY PETER COREY AND KARA MAY

Glossary

dribbly: melting, runny
clobber: slang for clothes
edible: safe to eat
appetite: a need or wish to eat

Understanding

1 Give **one** reason why chocolates might be a bad gift at the pictures.

2 Why is a wrestling magazine a bad gift for a boy to take to a girl's house?

3 Why does the author think perfume might be a good gift at the disco?

4 Is the advice on presents meant to be taken seriously? Give a reason for your answer.

5 All the good gifts are very predictable (stereotypical) gifts from males to females: chocolates, flowers, perfume. Think of **four** or **five** more unusual gifts that a boy might give a girl.

6 What are the stereotypical gifts girls are supposed to give to boys? Think of **four** or **five** creative (more unusual) alternatives.

Extended Writing

1 Copy and complete the following table.

Gifts from boys to girls		
Situation	Good gift	Bad gift
at the pictures	sweets	flowers
at a disco		
at the beach		
at the zoo		

2 Rewrite one section of the extract from the girl's point of view. For example, if a girl goes to the pictures with a boy, what would be a good/bad gift she could give him? Try to avoid stereotypical gifts. Try to make your advice funny, like the advice given in the extract.

Paragliding

By Kate Herbert

The closest thing to human flight, paragliding uses a hyper parachute and frame to ride the skies on thermal currents. Not to be confused with parascending (being towed into the sky by a speedboat or Land Rover) or hang-gliding.

How to do it

Find a recognized school and spend a week learning the basics to get your licence. You need a steep slope with the wind blowing up it – check with the landowner for permission – to take off, use air currents to stay up like a seagull against a cliff and steer by pulling the control toggles. Pull both toggles to slow down and land at your own pace.

Popularity

There are 9,000 members in the British Hang-gliding and Paragliding Association, of which around 7,000 are active paragliding pilots. About 6,000 others take a course each year.

Where to do it

Paragliders do it on hills and mountains. The three most popular areas in the UK are the South Downs, the Black Mountains in Wales, and the Peak District.

Contact for lessons

Call the British Hang-gliding and Paragliding Association (0116 261 1322) for details of local centres. A week's elementary pilot's course costs from £200, single lessons around £65 per day. A tandem flight costs around £35, for 10 minutes in the sky.

FROM **THE GUARDIAN**

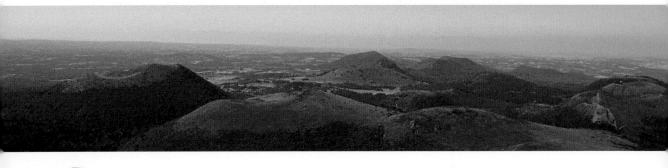

Glossary

hyper parachute: a specially-shaped parachute used for paragliding

thermal currents: air currents caused by warm air rising

recognized school: school or centre with qualified teachers/instructors

licence: a permit to do something, like fishing or driving

toggles: short pieces of wood/metal used as controls

elementary: beginners

tandem flight: two people (learner and instructor) on the same parachute

Understanding

1 How do you steer a paragliding parachute?
2 Where in Wales might you see paragliders in action?
3 How much would you expect to pay for a three-day course?
4 What is a tandem flight? Do you think it would be a dangerous thing to do? Give a reason for your answer.
5 Give **one** reason why weather forecasts are important for paragliders.

Extended Writing

1 Write a paragraph about the following **three** activities to show you understand how they are different from each other:
 • hang-gliding
 • paragliding
 • parascending.

Begin with this:

When you go hang-gliding you hang underneath a stiff wing in a special harness. Air currents lift the wing, and you, off the ground. You can steer the wing, just like steering a bike.

PF 22 2 Write a letter to the British Hang-gliding and Paragliding Association. Give details about yourself and say why you want to try paragliding. Tell them what course you would like to try and when you want to come. Ask them about paragliding centres near you. Ask also about dates, times, cost of courses, and whether you need insurance.

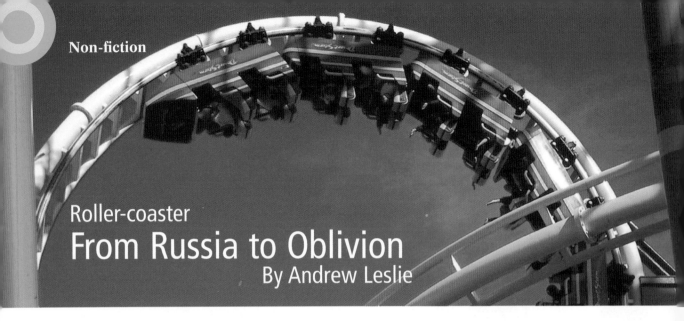

Roller-coaster
From Russia to Oblivion
By Andrew Leslie

The idea of the roller-coaster goes back centuries, but the real white-knuckle thrillers are only a few decades old.

1600s Ice slides constructed in a wooden framework in Russia. Climb the stairs and slide down.

1700s Slides using wheeled toboggans instead of ice appear in Europe. Called *Les montagnes Russes* (Russian mountains).

1874 In America, a gravity-powered coal-transport system is turned into a passenger-carrying 'scenic railway'.

1884 *Switchback Railways* installed in Coney Island, New York. The first real roller-coaster.

1900 Switchback designer John Miller patents 'upstops' – wheels running under the track to prevent cars lifting off at the top of hills. The roller-coaster suddenly becomes less 'tame'.

1920s The golden age of the American roller-coaster. 1,500 in operation worldwide. Built of wood, using the same techniques as for trestle bridges on American railroads.

1950s Walt Disney comes up with the idea of the theme park, and the roller-coaster gains a new popularity. Tubular steel is now used instead of wood.

1975 The first looping coaster appears.

1992 Construction of the first inverted coaster, when cars hang beneath the track rather than travel above it.

1998 Appearance of the first 'free-fall' roller-coaster, *Oblivion*.

FROM **CANDIS MAGAZINE**

Europe's Best Ride
By Paul Forster

The following were voted Europe's top five steel roller-coasters, in the European Coaster Club's 1998 survey:

1. **Nemesis**, 1994, Alton Towers, Staffordshire. Max G-force: 4; Track length: 716m; Max drop: 13m; Max speed: 81km/h

2. **The Big One**, 1994, Blackpool Pleasure Beach, Lancashire. Max G-force: 3.5; Track length: 1,665m; Max drop: 32m; Max speed: 136km/h

3. **Dragon Khan**, 1995, Universal's Port Aventura, Tarragona, Spain. Max G-force: 4; Track length: 1,285m; Max drop: 45m; Max speed: 110km/h

4. **Oblivion, 1998**, Alton Towers. Max G-force: 4.5; Track length: 373m; Max drop: 60m; Max speed: 110km/h

5. **Shockwave**, 1994, Drayton Manor, Staffordshire. Max G-force: 4; Track length: 500m; Max drop: 31m; Max speed: 80km/h

FROM THE **DAILY TELEGRAPH**

Glossary

decades: periods of ten years (e.g. the 1990s)
toboggans: small sledges used for sliding down hills
scenic: giving a fine view (e.g. a scenic route)
installed: built, put in place
golden age: a special time, the best time
trestle: wooden frame which holds something up, like scaffolding
inverted: turned upside down
free fall: dropping like a stone, pulled down by gravity

Understanding

1 In what year was the first real roller-coaster built?
2 What did John Miller invent? What effect did his invention have on roller-coasters?
3 What were roller-coasters made from in the 1920s? What new material was used in the 1950s?
4 What is an 'inverted' coaster?
5 How many years ago was the first looping roller-coaster made?
6 Which is the longest ride? Is this the longest ride in the world? Give a reason for your answer.
7 Which is the fastest ride? How fast does it go?
8 Which is the newest ride and where is it located?

Extended Writing

1 Use the information (opposite) to write a paragraph about one of Europe's best rides. For example, if you chose to write about Nemesis, you might begin like this:

The Nemesis was built in 1994, at Alton Towers, in the United Kingdom. When you ride on it you feel a maximum G-force of 4. The track is ...

PF 23 2 Carry out a survey of your group or class to find out what kinds of roller-coasters are the most popular with your age group, and why. Use this information to write a short article entitled 'White Knuckle Rides'.

Paragraph 1 Describe the kinds of rides which are most popular in your class.
Paragraph 2 Say what it is that people like about them.

Games Reviews

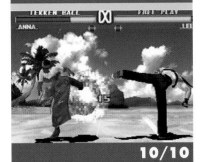

RENT OR BUY   COMING SOON

10/10

TEKKEN 3

Just when you thought 3D fighting games couldn't get any better, along come beat-'em-up experts Namco to prove us all wrong. The best 3D graphics you'll ever see in a virtual ruck combine with astonishing animated characters and limb-snapping moves in what has to be the world's finest ever beat-'em-up.

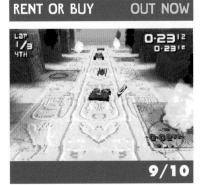

RENT OR BUY   OUT NOW

9/10

CIRCUIT BREAKERS

The most addictive and fun filled multi-player racing game yet to grace the PlayStation. Push your mates off the edge of the tracks and into devious traps as you race to the top of the championship. Great in one player, a certified classic in two, three or four.

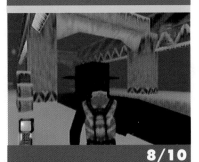

RENT OR BUY   SEPTEMBER

8/10

MISSION IMPOSSIBLE

Thought *GoldenEye 007* was a smasher? Then you'll absolutely love this. Tense spy action pushes you to the outer limits of gameplay as you struggle to overcome sneaky foreign plots and dirty domestic double-crossing in this action-packed 3D adventure.

FROM **THE SCENE** MAGAZINE

Glossary

3D: three dimensional
beat-'em-up: a type of video game in which the characters fight
ruck: fight
multi-player game: game played by more than one player
devious: sly
domestic: in your own country
double-crossing: cheating

Understanding

1 Which game can you rent or buy now?
2 Which game is not on sale until September?
3 Which game is given the highest score? Suggest one reason why it scored so highly.
4 What is the name of the company which makes *Tekken 3*?
5 If you liked *Golden Eye 007* which of the three new games does the reviewer think you will also enjoy?

Extended Writing

1 Read the three reviews again. Write down all the words and phrases used to persuade you to buy the games. Begin like this:

'The best 3D graphics you'll ever see'
'astonishing animated characters'

2 Use your list of words and phrases from Question 1 to write a review of a video game – real or invented. Say what type of game it is, who it will appeal to and why, and how it compares with other games.

wild, wet, and wonderful

Theme parks aren't the only places that are perfect for fun family breaks. Our superb collection of Center Parcs, Sunparks and Gran Dorado villages situated in France, Belgium, Holland, and Germany, guarantee year-round family fun that even the weather can't upset! Our wide array of Holiday Villages create a perfect haven for enjoyment, centered around a weather-proof dome housing a subtropical environment with swimming pools, water slides, saunas, and jacuzzis. It's not just indoor fun either, each village also offers a seemingly endless supply of outdoor activities ranging from wind surfing and sailing to mountain biking and archery. More than enough to satisfy even the most energetic family! Don't worry though, pure relaxation is also an option, just lazing around and enjoying a meal or a coffee at one of the restaurants and cafes are also popular activities.

Sunparks villages

Facilities	De Haan	Oostduinkerke	Vielsalm	Kempense Meren
Archery	●	●	●	●
Badminton	●	●	●	●
Basketball	●	●	●	●
Children's Pool	●	●	●	●
Crazy Golf	●	●	●	●
Cycling	●	●	●	●
Darts		●		
Sauna	●	●	●	●
Snooker	●	●	●	
Solarium	●	●		●
Squash	●	●	●	●
Table Tennis	●	●	●	●
Tennis Indoor/Outdoor	●	●	●	
Tenpin Bowling	●	●		●
Turkish Bath	●	●	●	●
Volleyball	●	●	●	●
Whirlpool	●	●		●

Gran Dorado villages

Facilities	Zandvoort	Port Zélande	Weerterbergen	Loohorst	Heilbachsee	Hochsauerland
Archery				●	●	●
Badminton	●	●	●	●	●	●
Basketball	●			●	●	
Bicycle Hire	●	●	●	●		●
Bowling	●	●	●	●	●	●
Canoeing	●	●	●	●		
Children's Pool	●	●	●	●	●	●
Darts	●	●	●	●	●	●
Mini-Golf	●		●	●	●	●
Mountain Bikes		●	●	●	●	
Sauna	●	●	●	●	●	●
Snooker	●		●	●		●
Solarium	●	●	●	●	●	
Squash	●	●	●	●		●
Table Tennis	●	●	●	●		●

Glossary

array: display, assortment, variety
haven: a shelter, a safe and peaceful place
subtropical: warm
saunas: steam-rooms (like a Turkish Bath)
jacuzzis: baths with underwater jets of water to massage the body
option: choice
facilities: activities on offer

Understanding

1 Name **two** Sunparks villages where you can play badminton.
2 At how many Gran Dorado villages can you hire a bike?
3 Name **one** activity you can enjoy at every village listed.
4 Is it true you can play snooker at most Sunparks villages? Give a reason for your answer.
5 Name **one** game you can play at all Gran Dorado villages, which is not available at any of the Sunparks villages.
6 Look at the facilities at Oostduinkerke and Loohorst. Which centre will be most popular with teenagers? Give a reason for your answer.

Extended Writing

1 Which village would you choose to visit? List the three activities you would most look forward to doing and say why. Begin like this:

I would chose to stay at … The three activities I would most look forward to doing are …

PF 24 **2** Carry out a survey in your group. Find out which facilities at Sunparks and Gran Dorado centres are the most popular. Also find out what other facilities the group would like that are not on offer at present.
Use this information to write a letter to a holiday company.
Paragraph 1   Describe which facilities, already on offer, are the most popular, and say why.
Paragraph 2   Suggest other activities which they might offer in future that will appeal to teenagers.

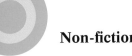

Thirties Child
Smacks and bed by 9.30

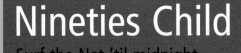

Nineties Child
Surf the Net 'til midnight

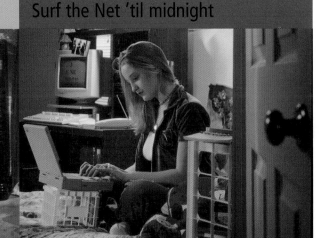

I WOULD be up at 7.30 to take a bowl of hot porridge to my father. After a 10-minute walk to my father's butcher's shop I would catch the bus to school.

At school things were very different from today. We all had to stand up when a teacher came into the room and we couldn't sit down until they said so.

Corporal punishment was used regularly. If you hadn't done your homework you'd be strapped. But the teachers usually kept order with a 3ft rule they used to slam down on your desk. We all sat up very straight in those days. School finished at 4pm.

Things were pretty tight, but my mother gave us the best she could provide, like a little corned beef. But never cheese, that was very tightly rationed.

After school finished, I would get the bus home and complete two hours of homework before father returned. All of us would then sit down for an evening meal.

If I behaved myself I was allowed to listen to the radio for a while before I went to bed at 9 or 9.30.

Ian Borland 73, of Shawlands, Glasgow

LIKE MOST people my age, an alarm clock is not enough. So, at seven every weekday, my human alarm clock, my mother, wakes me up.

At 7.35am I take my place at the 36 bus stop outside the Oval tube station. My school, The Grey Coat Hospital in Victoria, is only a mere 10 minutes away.

My day consists of seven 45-minute lessons. I spend my time swapping career ideas with my friend, Ebony, who encourages me, and we work together as a mini study group. We do this through phone calls, meetings, shopping, and general socializing.

Being a child of the technology era, my prized possession at the moment is my new mobile phone which comes in handy at lunch times when I can send messages to my friend when he's at college.

After a seven-and-a-half hour day which could easily pass for a lifetime, I return home. I spend the rest of my time watching *Neighbours, Home and Away* and *Jerry Springer*.

Then I surf the net and get my e-mails from friends. Sleep around midnight.

Juanita Rosenior 15, from London

FROM **THE INDEPENDENT** (ABRIDGED)

Glossary

corporal punishment: hitting with a cane or strap
pretty tight: money was short
socializing: meeting with, and talking to, friends
era: a period in history (e.g. the Victorian era)

Understanding

1 At what time did Ian Borland get up?
2 Where did he go on his way to school?
Why did he go there?
3 How was he punished at school if he misbehaved?
4 How much homework did he do?
5 How old is Juanita?
6 How long does it take her to get to school?
7 What does she talk about when she meets up with her friend, Ebony?
8 Why does Juanita say her seven-and-a-half hour day could 'pass for a lifetime'?

Extended Writing

1 If you could chose, would you be a 'Thirties Child', like Ian or a 'Nineties Child', like Juanita? Give reasons, and use information from the articles to support your answer.

2 When Juanita reads about Ian's childhood in the 1930s she decides to send him an e-mail. Write the e-mail. Try to write it in the style that Juanita is likely to use in an e-mail to her friends. It would be more casual than a formal letter. It might begin something like this:

Hi Ian! Just been reading about you and how things were the 1930s ...

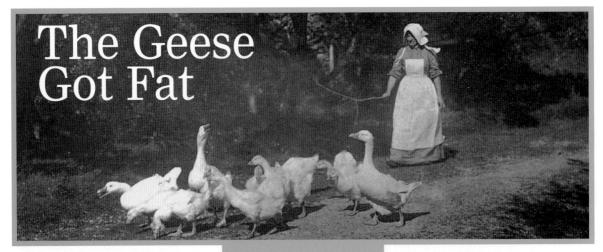

The Geese Got Fat

THE GEESE WERE then carried up to a room above the barn, the plucking room. After their day's work, our friends and neighbours came walking or riding horseback through the crisp-cold night air to help prepare the birds for market. This was considered the men's work. They clattered in their clogs up the stairs to the plucking room, seated themselves in a circle and began to pluck, the feathers being piled in the middle. You can imagine the joking, the exchange of news and the good fellowship of this friendly little community.

When the plucking was finished the birds were carried into the house and laid on the great stone poultry slab. This is where the ladies took over. They gathered up the feathers for cleaning and ultimate use in beds and cushions; then they fed their menfolk with a huge hot-pot followed by other delicacies, well laced with my mother's home-made wines of many varieties.

When the meal was over my father took each bird and immersed it, first in the

In this extract, Sarah Fisher recalls one memorable Christmas on her parents' Lancashire farm, in the 1890s. Her father reared 40 geese that year, which he killed two days before Christmas Day.

bubbling boiler by the roaring fire, and immediately out of this in icy cold water freshly drawn from the pump ... Next came the drawing and cleaning, and finally each bird, plump, white and neatly trussed, was ready for Preston Market. Only then did our friends leave, mostly to return to their neighbouring farms and start work with the first light.

At 5.30 am on Christmas Eve the trap was brought into the farmyard, freshly scrubbed from top to bottom. Then the goose cloths were brought out, snow-white sheets, reserved solely for the purpose and used only at Christmas. The first was laid on the trap floor, then came a layer of geese, covered by another cloth, and so on, until the trap was full and the final cloth tucked safely over them all.

Bess, the horse, was then brought out and harnessed to the trap. Mother stepped up, took the reins and off they went to Preston Market, the awesome distance of twelve miles.

Glossary

reared: brought up, raised from young

plucking: pulling the feathers off

clogs: heavy shoes with wooden soles

ultimate: final

hot-pot: a stew

delicacies: delicious foods

immersed: plunged into water

drawing: pulling out the innards

trussed: tied up

trap: small horse-drawn cart

harnessed: fastened

awesome: great, huge

Understanding

1 How many geese did Sarah's father rear?
2 Who helped her father to pluck the geese?
3 What were the feathers used for?
4 Which phrase tells you that Sarah's mother made different kinds of wine?
5 How were the geese taken to market?
6 What, in your own words, does to 'start work with the first light' mean?

Extended Writing

1 Read the extract again. Write down any information which gives you a clue about what life was like for Sarah in the 1890s. Begin like this:

Friends and neighbours helped each other.

They travelled on foot or horseback.

They wore clogs.

2 Imagine that Sarah appears in a time machine and takes you back to her Lancashire farm, and the year 1890. You spend Christmas Day with her and her family. Describe how you spend the day. Remember Sarah lives on a working farm, with no electricity, central heating or television! Try to use information from the list you made for Question 1. Begin like this:

Christmas Day

5.30 am. I help Sarah to feed the cows. The farmyard is slippery with ice. It is so dark we have to use a lantern to find our way from the farm house to the barn.

6 am. Get water from the pump. Try to wash. Icicles form on my nose!

111

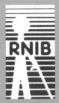

About RNIB

RNIB – Royal National Institute for the Blind – is Britain's largest organization working for blind and partially sighted people. It is one of the biggest and best known charities in the UK.

Facts and figures

More than one person in sixty in Britain is blind or partially sighted. That's almost a million people.

The majority of these are over the age of 60, as the chart below shows.

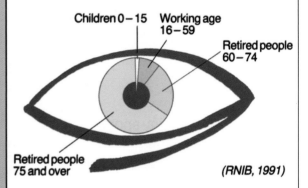

Children 0 – 15   Working age 16 – 59

Retired people 60 – 74

Retired people 75 and over

(RNIB, 1991)

In fact, one person in seven over the age of 75 has a severe visual impairment. And since most people now reach their 70s, that means there's roughly a one in seven chance any of us could develop serious sight problems.

Nearly three quarters of blind and partially sighted people are women.

Two thirds of the adults and a half of the children with impaired sight also have serious illness or disability.

Only a quarter of visually handicapped people of working age have jobs. Yet over half would like to work. With modern technology there are few jobs that they cannot do.

FROM **ABOUT RNIB**, AN INFORMATION LEAFLET PUBLISHED BY RNIB

Glossary

partially sighted: having some sight, not totally blind

majority: most people

impairment: something which may holds you back, stop you living life to the full

Understanding

1 What does RNIB stand for?
2 Which sentence tells you that a lot of people give money to the RNIB?
3 How many blind and partially sighted people are there in Britain?
4 Is it true that most of these people are old? Find a phrase to support your answer.
5 What percentage of visually handicapped people do not have a job?
6 What percentage would like a job?

Extended Writing

1 Copy and complete the following table.

Jobs blind people could do easily	Jobs which they might find difficult
author	airline pilot
tour guide	
music teacher	
physiotherapist	

2 The extract says: 'With modern technology there are few jobs blind and partially sighted people cannot do'. Write a letter to your local RNIB group, asking if someone could come along and talk to your group about this. Say what you would like the visitor to talk about. For example, you might want to know about how computers can help blind people. You will also have to include details about your class – the age of the students, the number in the group, the length of the lesson, etc.

Non-fiction

Will bungee-jumping push Nicholas Barber over the edge? Well, that's the general idea.

In the shadow of a 300ft crane – claimed to be the world's tallest bungee tower – I'm kitted out for my leap of faith. One harness loops through my legs and round my waist. An Australian fastens it pinchingly tight.

Another harness goes round both ankles, which are strapped together. This is no doubt an important safety measure, but I can't help thinking that its main purpose is to prevent me running away, as I am sorely tempted to do. As far as I can see, all that's missing is the inflatable crash mat which will cushion my fall when the rope snaps.

Then the Australian explains that the crash mat is already in place: it's

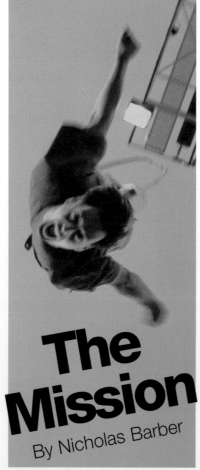

The Mission

By Nicholas Barber

called the river Thames.

I shuffle into the cage the size of a small lift – which is, in effect, what it is. The bungee rope is connected. Along for the ride are Graham, the Jump Master and another man with a camera on his shoulder, who is filming a souvenir video for me.

Within half a minute, the crane has winched us high above the rooftops of

London and swung us out over the river.

I can see the Millennium Dome in the distance. I wonder if I'll live to see its completion. Graham opens the gate.

I can't move. The Pepsi Max commercials were never like this. If you want to know how it feels to stand on a ledge, 300ft up, with a rubber band tied to your ankle, simply imagine standing on a ledge, 300ft up, *without* a rubber band tied to your ankle. Then I realize that if I hesitate now, my moment of shame will be recorded for ever on video. Vanity beats sanity, and I dive forward.

It's a rollercoaster times 10: fast, frightening, exhilarating, and supremely disorienting. 'You're not supposed to be this way up!' screams my instinct. I bounce half a dozen times as the crane swings over solid ground again and lowers the cage.

FROM THE **INDEPENDENT MAGAZINE** (ABRIDGED)

Glossary

sorely: very

crash mat: thick mat used to stop injury from a fall (e.g. in a gym)

souvenir: something you keep to remind you of a person, place or event

winched: hauled up by a crane

completion: finish

vanity: pride

sanity: common sense, reason

exhilarating: very exciting

supremely disorienting: leaves you not knowing where you are, which way you are facing, etc

instinct: something we do or feel without thinking

Understanding

1 How tall is the crane that Nicholas Barber jumps off?

2 Who is Graham?

3 Who else is in the cage with Nicholas? What does he do?

4 What can Nicholas see before he jumps?

5 Nicholas hesitates for a moment, then jumps. What, in your own words, makes him overcome his fear and jump?

6 What can he see as he falls through the air?

Extended Writing

1 Nicholas makes a joke about the straps around his ankles. What does he say? Who else makes a joke? What is this joke about?

2 You are a reporter like Nicholas Barber. You have been asked to write an article about bungee-jumping. You have to interview a number of people who have done bungee-jumps, to find out what is involved. Write down **five** or **six** questions which you would ask. Try not to ask closed questions – for example: 'Did you like it?' Try instead to ask open questions – for example: 'How did you feel before you jumped?' Think about asking questions that will give you information about equipment, safety, costs, as well as the feelings experienced by the bungee-jumper.

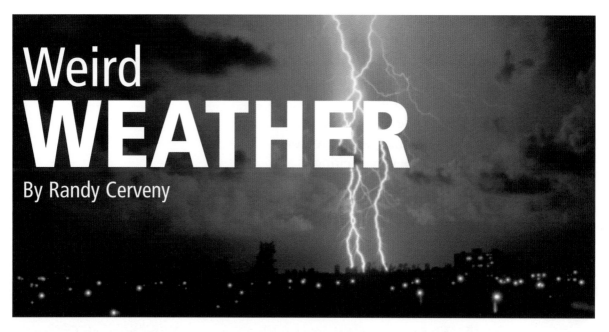

Weird
WEATHER

By Randy Cerveny

May 19, 1780

DARKNESS AT NOON: A smoky blackness settled over the New England states, possibly the result of massive forest fires in Western states. It was so dark that by noon, people had to light candles and lamps to see. Even with the aid of lanterns, farmers could scarcely get to their barns to care for their livestock.

May 29, 1892

EEL RAIN: An enormous number of eels fell during a rainstorm in Coalburg, [Alabama]. Farmers quickly drove into town with carts and took the eels away to use as fertilizer for their fields. The eel deluge – similar to other such peltings – may have resulted from a waterspout's lifting and jettisoning the fishes.

May 27, 1896

WAKE ME WHEN IT'S OVER: A massive tornado that hit the St Louis area picked up one sleeping resident along with his bed and mattress, carried him more than a quarter of a mile and left him unharmed – if unable to remember how he got there!

April 3, 1974

THE PICKY TORNADO: Despite demolishing an entire farmhouse in Xenia, Ohio, one of the worst tornadoes ever to hit the country left untouched a mirror, a case of eggs and a box of highly fragile Christmas ornaments.

July 9, 1995

NO SAFETY ANYWHERE: Lightning from a storm in Bristol, [Florida], struck a tree, sending a power surge through the water in a septic tank. The exploding water catapulted a 69-year-old man sitting on the toilet into the air. A hospital treated and released the man, who suffered only elevated blood pressure and tingling in his lower extremities.

FROM **SCIENTIFIC AMERICAN** MAGAZINE

Glossary

scarcely: hardly

deluge: downpour, flood

peltings: heavy rainfalls

waterspout: huge tube of water sucked up (from river or sea) by a tornado

jettisoning: throwing away

resident: someone who lives in that place

picky: choosey

fragile: easily broken

septic tank: tank which holds sewage and dirty water

elevated: raised

extremities: ends (of limbs)

Understanding

1 In what year was the sky in New England blotted out by black smoke?
2 Where and when did it rain eels?
3 What did the local farmers do with the eels?
4 How far was the sleeper from St Louis carried by the tornado?
5 Why is the 1974 Ohio tornado described as 'picky'?
6 How old was the man from Bristol, Florida?
7 What, in your own words, happened to him during the storm?

Extended Writing

1 Read the extract again. Decide which of the five incidents you think is the most frightening, and say why.

PF 25　2 Pick one of the five incidents. Imagine it happened in your street or neighbourhood. Write a short newspaper report using information from the extract, together with information about your local district. You will need to invent details such as dates, times, names, etc.

Tornado UK

The number of tornadoes reported in Britain has doubled in the past two years. What's going on?

Dakota lies in the heart of America's tornado country. Twisters spiral as if out of nowhere, razing towns and causing millions of dollars worth of damage. But at least the locals expect them.

In Britain, an average of 25 tornadoes are reported each year. This year there have been 25 reports in the first six months, with 18 in April alone.

Okay, so they don't cause the destruction that Mid-West residents have to put up with, but they can be pretty frightening.

A tornado that struck Reading [UK] recently crumbled bricks into rubble with ease. 'It was like something out of *The Wizard of Oz,*' said one observer.

So if tornadoes are on the increase, what's the cause?

Some experts are blaming global warming. In warmer weather, there's a greater tendency for tornadoes to form inland.

Professor Derek Elsom at Oxford Brookes University says the number of tornadoes hitting Britain has doubled in the past two years. But the Met Office isn't convinced that tornadoes are on the increase. 'More people do seem to be reporting them,' says a spokesman. 'But any time there's a strong wind associated with a thunderstorm, people tend to call it a tornado.'

FROM **FOCUS** MAGAZINE

Glossary

twisters: tornadoes
razing: destroying
Mid-West residents: people who live in the Mid-West states of the USA
global warming: increase in temperature of the Earth and its atmosphere
Met Office: the Meteorological Office, a government department which studies and reports on the weather
convinced: sure, certain

Understanding

1 Which place in America is at the centre of tornado country?
2 How many tornadoes are reported in Britain in an average year?
3 Which sentence tells you that tornadoes in the USA are more powerful than those in Britain?
4 If the number of tornadoes is increasing, what might be the cause?

Extended Writing

1 Not everyone is sure that the number of tornadoes hitting Britain is increasing. There are two different views put forward in the article. One is put forward by Professor Elsom. The other is put forward by a spokesman from the Met Office. Read the last two paragraphs of the article again. Then write two sentences to show you understand the difference between these two views. Begin the sentences like this:

Professor Elsom believes that …

The spokesman from the Met Office disagrees with the professor because he thinks …

PF 26 2 In the book *The Wizard of Oz*, the heroine, Dorothy, is carried off by a violent tornado to the strange land of Oz.

Write the opening section of a fantasy story in which the main character – a young person – is carried away by a tornado and lands in a very strange place. Describe what it would be like to be blown thousands of feet into the air, spinning round like a top. What kind of noises would you hear? What else would get carried away with you?

SNARRI THE JEWELLER

**SNARRI WORKS
AS A JEWELLER
IN VIKING YORK.**

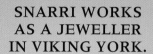

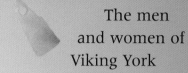

In Viking York both men and women wear much more jewellery than we do today. Men wear brooches shaped like a disc which are used to fasten cloaks. Pendants, finger-rings and arm-rings are also worn. Belts have elaborate buckles and strap ends and swords and knives have ornate metal mounts. Women wear similar jewellery with the addition of earrings and strings of beads.

Jewellery is made of copper, lead, silver, and gold; even glass is made into finger-rings. Amber and jet are commonly made into jewellery in Jorvik workshops.

The men and women of Viking York look gaudy to modern eyes – wearing their brightly coloured clothes and glittering jewels. They even have tattoos. They wear red, yellow, purple, blue, and green clothes edged with coloured braids. Men wear long-sleeved tunics and trousers. Beneath the tunic is a linen shirt and over all is a heavy cloak of fur or cloth. Women wear long dresses over which a length of cloth with shoulder straps is wrapped around the body under the arms. Shawls keep them warm, and small silk caps are worn on the head.

FROM THE OFFICIAL GUIDEBOOK OF THE
JORVIK VIKING CENTRE, YORK

Glossary

pendants: jewellery worn around the neck on a cord or chain
elaborate: fancy
ornate: having a lot of decoration
amber: a hard, yellow material used to make jewellery
jet: a hard, black mineral
gaudy: showy, brightly coloured
braids: strips of different coloured cloth woven into a plait
tunics: jackets
linen: cloth made from flax (a plant)

Understanding

1 Where does Snarri the jeweller work?
2 Name the **seven** materials that Snarri uses to make jewellery.
3 What, in your own words, does the following mean: 'The men and women of Viking York look gaudy to modern eyes'?
4 What do Viking men wear over their tunics?
5 Why do Viking women wear shawls?

Extended Writing

1 Read the extract again. Make a list of the main differences between the way Vikings dress and the way we dress today. Begin like this:

Viking men and women wear more jewellery than we do.
Viking men wear swords and knives.
Viking clothes are more brightly coloured than ours.

2 If Snarri the jeweller could travel in time and visit you in your home, how would he react to the clothes you wear? What would he say about zips, stretch fabrics (like Lycra), designer trainers, and school uniform? Write a dialogue between you and Snarri in which you talk about some of your favourite clothes. You might start like this:

Snarri: What is this called?
You: It's a T-shirt.
Snarri: What is it made from?
You: Cotton.

Ferry Sinks in Shark Hell

Lindsay Oakley and Caroline Pook were on a ferry in the Pacific Ocean, off the coast of Fiji, when it sank.

Lindsay's story

Behind us, people were panicking and jostling for lifejackets. The cabin rapidly filled with water. The last person crawled out, and the boat rolled over. It had all happened in just three minutes.

And there we were – 23 helpless souls, bobbing around our capsized boat, miles from anywhere.

A horrible burning sensation spread over my chest and stomach, we could all feel it – petrol burns from the leaking engines.

Some people were crying. Some didn't have lifejackets – there were only 16 for 23 of us. We heaved the non-swimmers on to the upturned hull; the rest of us trod water, clinging to whatever we could.

The captain tried to reassure us. 'People will come when we don't reach Lautoka,' he said. But that wasn't the first of my concerns.

My fears were with what might be lurking beneath the surface, perhaps right at this minute. Every one of us knew these seas were infested with sharks but, like an unspoken code, no one mentioned them. So far we hadn't seen any of the dreaded tell-tale fins – but that didn't mean they hadn't seen us.

Hour after hour we clung there, freezing cold despite the intense sun. At one point, we saw a cruise liner in the distance. The captain dived into the cabin, and emerged with a flare. 'Please see us,' we all prayed, but the flare didn't go high enough. The liner glided silently away.

By 4.30pm, we knew we had to do something – it would be dark in another couple of hours and the boat was slowly, but surely, sinking. 'The nearest island is at least an hour's swim away,' said the captain. We discussed it amongst ourselves.

'I'll swim,' said an English girl I now know as Caroline. 'Me, too,' said Olivia. 'I'll stay here, to help the non-swimmers and those without lifejackets,' I said.

After much debate, 13 swam off, leaving 10 of us clinging to the upturned boat.

'See you soon, okay?' I said to Olivia. But would I ever see her again?

We watched until they were just dots on the horizon.

As night fell, the water became more choppy – waves washed over us, knocking us into the water. Each time, it became harder to climb back on to the hull.

For the first time I began to doubt we'd make it. Two more cruise ships sailed by, their lights blazing in the darkness. There was no way we'd be rescued now.

(continued on page 126)

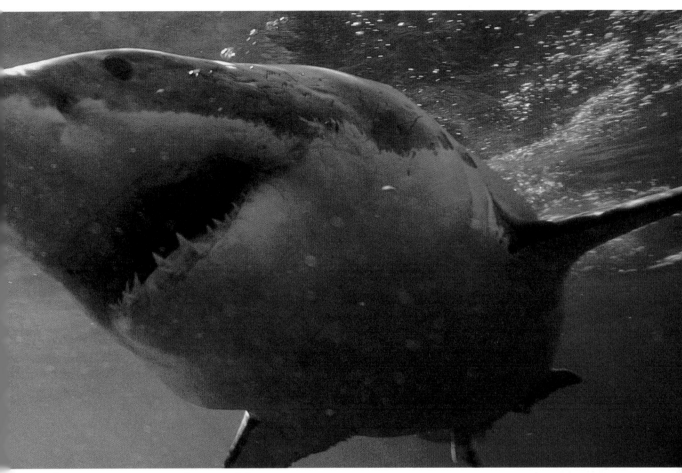

Glossary

jostling: pushing
capsized: turned over
lurking: waiting nearby, unseen
infested: full of
intense: very strong
debate: discussion, argument
hull: the main part of the ship, which holds the passengers or cargo
choppy: rough

Understanding

1 How long did it take for the boat to roll over?
2 How many people escaped from the capsized boat?
3 How many people did not have lifejackets?
4 Where was the ferry going when it capsized?
5 How do you know Lindsay is a good swimmer?
6 What happened to make Lindsay think they would not be rescued?

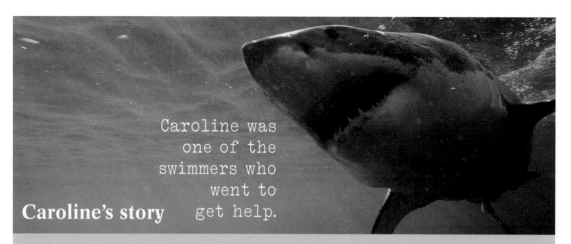

Caroline was one of the swimmers who went to get help.

Caroline's story

After two hours I was exhausted, but we swam on. I was holding the hand of a New Zealand girl, Olivia, making sure she didn't fall behind.

'We'll be swimming in the dark soon,' I fretted as the sun set. But there was a more frightening thought lurking in the back of my mind. Night was feeding time for sharks. Would any of us survive until dawn?

We formed a huddle to rest, and clung on to each other, literally, for dear life. Our limbs screamed in protest as we struck out again into the inky darkness.

We were on the point of collapse, when someone shouted: 'What's that over there?'

In the gloom we could just make out an island. I was the first to it, hauling myself onto the rocks with my last dregs of energy. We'd been swimming a solid four hours. We all collapsed, exhausted, onto a patch of sand.

As we huddled there, trying to ignore our searing dehydration headaches, Cory said: 'You know, I saw a shark fin earlier on, just before it got dark. I thought it best not to say anything'.

'I saw it too,' said the French guy. A chill ran over my already goosebumped flesh.

We fell silent, praying for the others still clinging to the almost submerged boat.

'A light!' someone suddenly whispered. It was 3.30am and a ship's searchlight was beaming across the sea at us. I burst into tears. Had they seen us? I fished my wet torch out of my bum bag and flashed it in reply.

Shortly after dawn, the ship turned towards us. When it came close, we recognized the faces of the people we'd left on the boat – now waving frantically. I sobbed with joy. It turned out we'd been saved by a miracle of fate – no one had been searching for us. By chance the capsized boat had drifted towards a cruiseship in the night. Passengers who heard shouts from the sea alerted the crew.

We were bedraggled and exhausted. All our possessions were sitting on the bottom of the sea – but we felt like we had the world.

FROM **BELLA** MAGAZINE

Glossary

fretted: worried

huddle: a small group

limbs: arms and legs

dregs: worthless or last bits (as in the dregs in the bottom of a barrel)

searing: very painful

dehydration: lack of water

submerged: below the water

alerted: told, warned

bedraggled: untidy, wet, and dirty

Understanding

7 Why did Caroline hold Olivia's hand?

8 Give **two** reasons why Caroline started to worry as night fell.

9 Who saw the shark fins? Why didn't they tell the other swimmers until later?

10 When did the swimmers first see the rescue boat? When were they finally rescued?

11 Why, in your own words, did Caroline say 'we felt like we had the world'?

Extended Writing

1 Make a chart like this to show the dangers faced by Lindsay and Caroline. Then tick the boxes to show which woman experienced which danger.

Danger	Lindsay	Caroline
Being trapped in the ferry when it capsized		
Petrol burns		
Sharks		

2 When Lindsay and Caroline meet up after their ordeal, Lindsay wants to know what happened to Caroline and the other swimmers, when they swam off to get help. Re-read Caroline's story. Pick out the most important parts of her account and write a summary. Write it as a first person narrative, using 'I' and 'we'. Begin like this:

We swam for two hours. By then I was very tired. Then it started to get dark. I was pretty scared because ...

Acknowledgements

The author and publisher are grateful for permission to reprint copyright material:

John Agard: 'One Question from a Bullet' from *Mangoes and Bullets* (Pluto Press, 1985), reprinted by kind permission of John Agard c/o Caroline Sheldon Literary Agency; **David Almond**: extract from *Kit's Wilderness* (Hodder Children's Books, 1999), reprinted by permission of Hodder & Stoughton Ltd; **K A Applegate**: extract from *Animorphs 1: The Invasion* (1992), copyright © 1992 by K A Applegate, reprinted by permission of the publishers, Scholastic, Inc.; **Andrea Ashworth**: extract from *Once in a House on Fire* (Picador, 1998), reprinted by permission of Macmillan; **Nicholas Barber**: extracts from 'The Mission', *The Independent Magazine*, 16.1.99, reprinted by permission of the Independent; **Valerie Bloom**: 'Haircut Rap' from *Let Me Touch the Sky* (Macmillan Children's Books, 2000), reprinted by permission of the author; **Betsy Byars**: *The House of Wings* (Bodley Head), reprinted by permission of the Random House Group Ltd; **Michele Celeste**: extracts from *Mariza's Story* (Heinemann, 1994), reprinted by permission of Heinemann Educational Publishers, a division of Reed Educational & Professional Publishing Ltd.; **Randy Cerveny**: extracts from 'It's Raining Eels: A Compendium of Weird Weather', from *Scientific American Presents Weather: What We Can and Can't Do About It*, Spring 2000, copyright © 2000 Scientific American, Inc, all rights reserved, reprinted by permission of Scientific American, Inc; **Sandra Cisneros**: 'Good Hot Dogs' from *My Wicked Wicked Ways*, (published by Alfred A Knopf 1989, originally published in paperback by Third Woman Press), copyright © 1987 by Sandra Cisneros, reprinted by permission of Susan Bergholz Literary Services, New York. All rights reserved; **Peter Corey**: extract from *Coping With Girls* (Scholastic Ltd, 1992), reprinted by permission of the publisher; **Roald Dahl and Richard R George**: extract from *Charlie and the Chocolate Factory: A Play* (Puffin, 1979), reprinted by permission of David Higham Associates; **Fred D'Aguiar**: 'Mama Dot', © Fred D'Aguiar 1985, from *Mama Dot* (Chatto & Windus, 1985), reprinted by permission of David Higham Associates; **Narinder Dhami**: extract from *Annie's Game* (Corgi Yearling, a division of Transworld Publishers, 1999), copyright © Narinder Dhami 1999, reprinted by permission of the publishers. All rights reserved; **Sarah Fisher**: extract from 'The Geese Got Fat' in *A Lancashire Christmas* compiled by John Hudson (Sutton, 1990), originally published in *Lancashire Life*, 1972; copyright holder not traced; **Paul Forster**: 'Europe's Best Rides' extract from 'White Knuckle Rides', *Daily Telegraph* 29.7.99, reprinted by permission of the Telegraph Group Ltd; **Sarah Forsyth**: 'My Christmas – Mum's Christmas' from 'A Child's View of Christmas' in *Glitter When You Jump* edited by Helen Exley, copyright © Exley Publications Ltd 1979, reprinted by permission of the publisher; **H B Gilmour**: extract from *Godzilla* (Puffin, 1998), from the screenplay by Dean Devlin and Roland Emmerich, copyright © Tristar Pictures Inc, 1998, reprinted by permission of The Copyright Promotions Licensing Group PLC. 'Godzilla' and 'Baby Godzilla' and the Godzilla character designs are trademarks and copyrights of Toho Co Ltd, 1998. All Rights Reserved; **David Harmer**: 'Watch Your Teacher Carefully', copyright © David Harmer 1995, first published in John Foster and Korky Paul: *Monster Poems* (OUP, 1995), reprinted by permission of the author; **Kate Herbert**: extracts from 'Paragliding', *The Guardian* 21.2.97, copyright © The Guardian 1997, reprinted by permission of The Guardian; **Paul Jennings**: extract from *Unmentionable* (Puffin, 1992), reprinted by permission of the publisher, Penguin Books Australia Ltd; **Sarah Kennedy** (ed): extracts by Clive Kavanagh, Barbara Godfrey and Win and Neil Morley from *The Terrible Twos: True Stories of Tots and Toddlers* (BBC), compilation copyright © Sarah Kennedy, copyright in the individual pieces rests with the contributors, reprinted by permission of BBC Worldwide Limited; **Bernard Kops**: extract from *Dreams of Anne Frank* (1992), reprinted by permission of David Higham Associates; **Fran Landesman**: 'Crying to Get Out' from *Golden Handshake* by Fran Landesman (1981), reprinted by permission of Jay Landesman; **Tom Leonard**: 'Boy, 9, rides 150 miles under lorry', *Daily Telegraph* 5.11.97, reprinted by permission of the Telegraph Group Ltd; **Andrew Leslie**: 'From Russia to Oblivion' extract from 'White Knuckle Terror', from August 1998 issue of *Candis*, the best selling monthly family magazine published by Newhall Publications. *Candis* helps raise over £1.5 million for medical charities each year. For more information ring Norman Firkins on 0151 632

7648; **Christobel Mattingley**: extract from *No Gun for Asmir* (Penguin, 1993), reprinted by permission of the publisher, Penguin Books Australia Ltd; **Michael Morpurgo**: extract from *The Wreck of the Zanzibar* (Heinemann Young Books, an imprint of Egmont Children's Books Ltd, London, 1995), copyright © Michael Morpurgo 1995, reprinted by permission of the publishers and David Higham Associates; extract from *War Horse* (Kaye & Ward 1982), copyright © Michael Morpurgo 1982, reprinted by permission of Egmont Children's Books Ltd, London; **Cherry Norton**: 'Smacks and bed by 9.30' (Thirties Child) and 'Surf the Net 'til midnight' (Nineties Child), *The Independent* 2.9.99, reprinted by permission of The Independent; **Clifford Oliver**: extract from *Sitting Pretty* (ARC Theatre Publications, 1999), reprinted by permission of the publishers, ARC Theatre Publications, Kingsmoor Lodge, Paringdon Road, Harlow, Essex CM19 4QT, from whom the full script can be obtained; **Philip Ridley**: extract from *The Meteorite Spoon* (Viking, 1994), copyright © Philip Ridley 1994, reprinted by permission of Penguin Books Ltd and A P Watt Ltd on behalf of the author; **Jamie Rix**: extract from 'Glued to the Telly' in *Grizzly Tales for Gruesome Kids* by Jamie Rix (Scholastic Ltd), reprinted by permission of the publisher; **Richard Robinson**: 'Cool Spoons' from *Conjuring in the Kitchen* (OUP, 1999), reprinted by permission of Oxford University Press. **Hal Summers**: 'The Rescue', copyright © Hal Summers 1962, from Charles Causley (ed): *Dawn to Dusk* (Brockhampton Press, 1962), reprinted by permission of the author; **Victoria Wood**: 'Supermarket Checkout' from *Chunky* (Methuen, 1996), reprinted by permission of the publisher; **Edmond Leo Wright**: 'I would Run with My Shadow' from *Over the Bridge* an anthology of new poems edited by John Loveday (Puffin 1981), copyright holder not traced; and also
Attic Futura for extracts from 'Your Shout!' in *Sugar*, March 2000; **H Bauer Publishing** and the authors for 'Behind the Headlines', Lindsay's story by Robin Corry, and Caroline's story by Janet Hawkins from *Bella* 37, 14.9.99; **Blockbuster Entertainment Ltd** and **Future Publishing Ltd** for game reviews for *Tekken 3* (Sony), *Circuit Breakers* (Mindscape) and *Mission Impossible* (Infogrames) from issue 7 (August 1998) of Blockbuster's in-house magazine, *The Scene*; **Bridge Travel Service** for extracts from *Go Wild* brochure for Holidays at European Theme Parks, 1999; **The National Magazine Company Ltd** for 'Tornado UK', adapted from *Focus*, June 1998, © National Magazine Company; **Ross Parry News and Picture Agency** for 'Son Saves Sick Father' as published by *The Daily Mirror*, 28.11.98; **RNIB** for extracts from brochure 'About RNIB'; **RSPCA** for 'Animal Hospital' diary from *Animal Hospital*, June/July 2000; **D C Thomson & Co Ltd** for extract from 'I was Haunted by the Internet' from *Shout Magazines Scary Stories* (D C Thomson, 1998); **Walker Books Ltd**, London for extract from 'Ears, Eyes, Legs and Arms' collected by Ced Hesse and told to him by Mamdou Karambe, and illustration by Louise Brierley, from *South & North, East & West* edited by Michael Rosen, edited text © Michael Rosen 1992, illustrations © Louise Brierley 1992; **Well Worth Reading** for reviews of 'Vampire Stories to tell in the dark' first published in *BOOX* Magazine, Well Worth Reading, issue 2; **York Archaeological Trust for Excavation and Research Ltd** for extract from Jorvik Viking Centre *Official Guidebook*, 1999.

Although every effort has been made to trace and contact copyright holders before publication this has not been possible in some cases. If notified the publisher will be pleased to rectify any errors or omissions at the earliest opportunity.

Photograph Credits
p.6 Digital Vision; p.8 Getty Images/Robert Holmgren; p.10 Corel; p.12 John Walmsley; p.14 Corbis/Tim Page (bottom), PA Photos (top); p.16 Corel; p.18 Lego; p.20 Hulton; p.22 Getty Images/Bob Torrez; p.24 Oxford Scientific Films/Deni Bown; p.26 Mary Evans Picture Library; p.28 Illustration by Louise Brierley; p.32 Martin McKenna; p.36 Digital Vision; p.40 Getty Images/Garry Hunter; p.42 Getty Images/Andrew Hall; p.46 Corel (top), Digital Vision (bottom); p.48 Mary Evans Picture Library; p.50 Getty Images/ Brian Bailey; p.52 Corel; p.54 Image Bank/ Jody Dole; p.56 Corel; p.58 Corbis/Gary W. Carter; p.60 Corel; p.68 Corbis/Thomas Brummett; p.72 Corbis/Bettmann; p.74 Digital Vision; p.78 Getty Images/Sue Cunningham; p.80 Corel; p.86 Corel; p.88 RSPCA/Tim Sambrook; p.98 Corel; p.100 Getty Images/Hubert Camille; p.102 Corel; p.106 Corel; p.108 Telegraph Colour Library /FPG International (left), Getty Images/Andy Sacks (right); p.110 Hulton; p.114 Getty Images/Charles Thatcher; p.116 Corel; p.120 Corbis/Jim Zuckerman; p.120 York Archaeological Trust; p.124 Getty Images /Chuck Davis.